Clinical Management of Breastfeeding

Clinical Management of Breastfeeding

Anil Mokashi MD DCH FIAP PhD (Pediatrics)
Consultant Pediatrician
Baramati, Maharashtra, India

Santosh Nimbalkar MBBS DCH
Consultant Pediatrician
Kolhapur, Maharashtra, India

Foreword
Arun Gupta

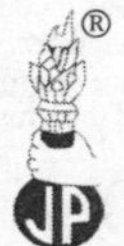

JAYPEE BROTHERS MEDICAL PUBLISHERS (P) LTD

New Delhi • London • Philadelphia • Panama

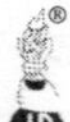

Jaypee Brothers Medical Publishers (P) Ltd

Headquarters

Jaypee Brothers Medical Publishers (P) Ltd
4838/24, Ansari Road, Daryaganj
New Delhi 110 002, India
Phone: +91-11-43574357
Fax: +91-11-43574314
Email: jaypee@jaypeebrothers.com

Overseas Offices

J.P. Medical Ltd
83 Victoria Street, London
SW1H 0HW (UK)
Phone: +44-2031708910
Fax: +44-(0)20-3008-6180
Email: info@jpmedpub.com

Jaypee-Highlights Medical Publishers Inc.
City of Knowledge, Bld. 237, Clayton
Panama City, Panama
Phone: + 507-301-0496
Fax: + 507-301-0499
Email: cservice@jphmedical.com

Jaypee Brothers Medical Publishers Ltd
The Bourse
111 South Independence Mall East
Suite 835, Philadelphia, PA 19106, USA
Phone: + 267-519-9789
Email: joe.rusko@jaypeebrothers.com

Jaypee Brothers Medical Publishers (P) Ltd
17/1-B Babar Road, Block-B, Shaymali
Mohammadpur, Dhaka-1207
Bangladesh
Mobile: +08801912003485
Email: jaypeedhaka@gmail.com

Jaypee Brothers Medical Publishers (P) Ltd
Shorakhute, Kathmandu
Nepal
Phone: +00977-9841528578
Email: jaypee.nepal@gmail.com

Website: www.jaypeebrothers.com
Website: www.jaypeedigital.com

Inquiries for bulk sales may be solicited at: jaypee@jaypeebrothers.com

Clinical Management of Breastfeeding

First Edition: **2013**

ISBN : 978-93-5090-349-0

Printed at Rajkamal Electric Press, Plot No. 2, Phase-IV, Kundli, Haryana.

Dedicated to

Late Dr Madhav Eknath Mokashi. He said,
"Spend your time and energy in doing good. Money follows."

Dedicated to

Foreword

More than 18 years back, a famous cardiothoracic surgeon whom I went to see for the surgery of my father-in-law, asked me, "What is your specialty?" I answered, "Human lactation management." He was pleasantly surprised and said, "This was unheard of."

The book *Clinical Management of Breastfeeding* by Dr Anil Mokashi and Dr Santosh Nimbalkar presents a sound thinking that health workers and professionals need to spend time in gaining skills to manage human lactation. It makes a point. Lactation management is the need of all health systems.

We have come a long way but still miles to go!

The book clearly lays emphasis on building skilled breastfeeding or infant and young child feeding counselors. This is necessary for all health facilities, public or private. Women who come to deliver in health facilities trust health workers/ professionals, therefore, it is highly justified that they acquire the knowledge and skills that are needed to make a woman successful in breastfeeding within one hour and maintain exclusive breastfeeding for the first 6 months.

Several chapters of the book deal with different and varied issues including how to talk to a mother, how to take history and dealing with low birth weight babies makes it special. The chapter dealing with production and intake of breast milk is critical for success as is the understanding that breastfeeding is a process determined by hormonal control and dependent on sucking by the baby. Chapter on inadequate milk gives a view to deal with this issue with utmost care as this is just a symptom of a problem, which needs investigation and more of perceived risk than real. Expressing breast milk is another important skill to be learnt by all health workers and women who come for delivery.

The book clearly underlines the need for skill building of health workers and counselors for breastfeeding and infant and young child feeding counseling. Coupled with the knowledge that it provides in easy, readable and understandable manner, this can be a useful resource to prevent and manage problems of breastfeeding and especially when women perceive that they do not have enough milk for their babies. It can give confidence to its readers who can then build the confidence of mothers; the most critical link if broken, leads to failure of breastfeeding or adoption of artificial feeding.

Needless to say, the book will make an important addition to the education materials for lactation management in health systems.

I hope this kind of curriculum gets into all medical and nursing studies both in theory and clinical practice. All health workers who deal with women and children must get this kind of knowledge and skills.

Arun Gupta MD (Pediatrics) FIAP
Central Coordinator
Breastfeeding Promotion Network of India
Regional Coordinator
International Baby Food Action Network (IBFAN) Asia
New Delhi, India

Preface

Mother's milk, or human milk, is the biggest, richest, most precious untapped natural asset. It is unadulterated and 'ready-to-eat' food. It is species specific, created by nature for human babies. We need plans or schemes at national, state, local, family and individual levels, to utilize 'human milk' as a national resource. Unfortunately, breastfeeding promotion is left to a handful of activists.

There is a massive lack of trained manpower in this field. "Professional, Practicing Lactation Management Counselors" is a social need of the nation. Few doctors know the science of lactation and breastfeeding. Still few have practised the art. Qualified doctors, busy in curative practice, take breastfeeding lightly. They are not serious, responsible, accountable and committed to breastfeeding.

Unfortunately, lactation management has no place in 'any educational curriculum'. Educated families also make grave mistakes, leading to lactation failure, affecting growth and development of child/infant population. Lactation failure is not a disease to be cured by drugs. The people and actions against natural process of lactation leads to lactation failure. Lactation is a matter of confidence. It is the people around who can increase or decrease it.

Lactation management counselors are trained to: (1) Handle lactation problems, (2) Motivate families to have a positive approach, (3) Visit the mother in hospital on the day of delivery, (4) Enquire about pregnancy, delivery and previous lactation experience, (5) Examine the breasts and the baby, (6) Observe the breastfeed and (7) Guide if there is any problem.

It is not essential to be a doctor to become a lactation management counselor. Pediatricians, gynecologists, doctors, physiotherapists, clinical psychologists, naturopaths, dietitians, home science graduates, their wives or close relatives can pursue this career. This book is designed for Lactation Management Counselors (LMCs). Thanks to innumerable sources we have drawn from!

Anil Mokashi
Santosh Nimbalkar

Acknowledgments

I would like to thank:

- My co-author, Dr Santosh Nimbalkar, for his patience and perseverance.
- My wife, Dr Madhuri Mokashi, for all the help.
- Dr Ashutosh Joshi, for academic exercises behind this script.
- Reva Mokashi, for the help with her English language editing expertise.
- Shri Jitendar P Vij (Group Chairman), Mr Ankit Vij (Managing Director) and Mr Tarun Duneja (Director-Publishing) of M/s Jaypee Brothers Medical Publishers (P) Ltd, New Delhi, India, for taking up the noble cause.

—Anil Mokashi

I am grateful to all those who helped me in writing this book. First of all, I would like to thank Dr Anil Mokashi, my co-author, who encouraged me. He had immense faith and belief in my devotion towards the subject. I would also like to thank my colleagues who supported me. I thank my brother, Professor Dr Somashekhar Nimbalkar, Eminent Teacher and Pediatrician, who has been a constant support and guide to me. My wife, Dr Sangeeta Nimbalkar, has been my greatest critic and support to me. The blessings of my parents has made this endeavor a success. Lastly, I express my gratitude towards patients, mothers and babies, whose need has inspired to write this book.

—Santosh Nimbalkar

Acknowledgements

[illegible]

- My co-author Dr. Sa[illegible] [illegible]
- [illegible]
- [illegible]
- [illegible]

— [illegible] Moksh[illegible]

I am [illegible] First of all [illegible] Dr. Anil [illegible] [illegible] Eminent Teacher and Paediatrician [illegible] support [illegible] to me [illegible] this book.

— [illegible] Nimbalkar

Contents

chapter 1

Lactation, Breastfeeding and Infant Feeding

Exclusive Breastfeeding

Exclusive breastfeeding means giving a baby no other food or drink including water, in addition to breastfeeding with the exception of syrup or drops of vitamins, minerals and medicines (expressed breast milk is also permitted) (Fig. 1.1).

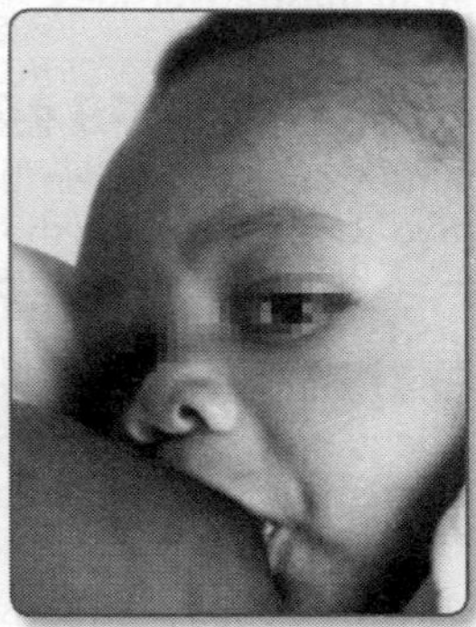

Fig. 1.1: Breastfeeding: perfect

Predominant Breastfeeding

Baby requires breast milk as the predominant source of nourishment and allows the infant to receive liquids (water or water-based drinks, fruit juice).

Complementary Feeding

Infant receives breast milk along with solid and semisolid foods.

Partial Breastfeeding

It means giving a baby some breastfeeds and some artificial feeds, either milk or cereals or other foods.

Bottle Feeding

Feeding the baby from bottle, whatever is in the bottle, including expressed breast milk.

Breastfeeding and Low Birth Weight Babies

Breast milk of mothers of low birth weight babies has higher concentration of proteins, essential fatty acids and sodium which is more suitable for them. Preterm babies need extra-protection from cold, infections and metabolic derangement. They have more chances of growth failure and necrotizing enterocolitis. Breastfeeding protects low birth weight babies from these adversities.

Breastfeeding and Malnutrition

Fifty percent children below 3 years are malnourished. In two-thirds, it starts in the first year of life. Children are anemic, have vitamins A and D deficiency. Starvation causes 60% of under-5 deaths. Most of these deaths are due to diarrhea and pneumonia. Exclusive breastfeeding up to 6 months and adequate complementary feedings along with breastfeeding thereafter reduces undernutrition, anemia and vitamin deficiencies. In affluent society, 15% children are overweight and a large number of them are obese. Breastfeeding prevents children being obese too.

Breastfeeding and Cognitive Development (Knowledge-based Development)

The effect is seen in infancy, childhood up to 15 years. Breastfed babies have 5–8 higher intelligence quotient (IQ) points than animal milk-fed babies (Figs 1.2A and B). Other proven advantages are visual maturation, language development,

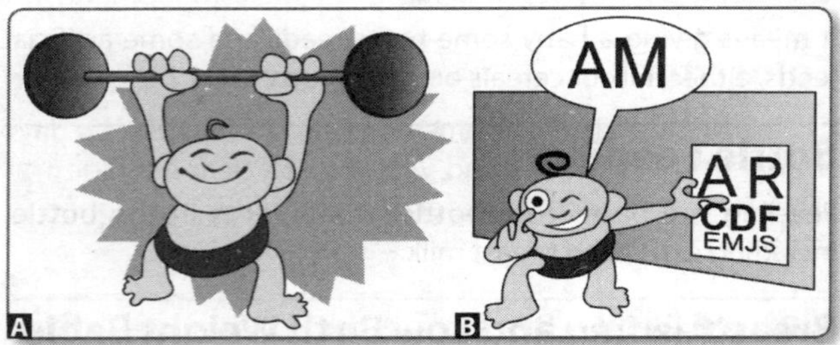

Figs 1.2A and B: (A) Body exercise builds body; (B) Brain exercise builds brain

fewer emotional or behavior problems, less aggressive personality and fewer minor neurological problems.

Risk of not Breastfeeding

Infants who are not breastfed, and receive formula milk or other replacement feeds have: (i) sixfold increased risk of dying in the first 2 months of life, (ii) fourfold increased risk of dying between 2 and 3 months and (iii) twofold to fivefold increased risk of dying between 4 and 5 months, compared with those who are breastfed. Breastfeeding in the first 6 months of life substantially reduces deaths from diarrhea and acute respiratory infections. Two-thirds of infant deaths occur in the first 2 months of life. When the mother is infected, white cells in mother's body produce antibodies which are secreted in the breast milk to protect the baby.

Advantages of Proper Complementary Feeding

The young child should be made accustomed to eating family foods. Complementary feeding should be started when the baby can no longer get enough energy and nutrient from breast milk alone. For most babies, this is after 6 months of age. If young children do not have enough good food, they will not have energy to grow and be active. Adequate complementary feeding prevents undernutrition, anemia, vitamin deficiencies, illnesses, and promotes proper growth and development.

Colostrum

It is the breast milk that women produce in the first few days after delivery. It is thick and yellowish or clear in color. The properties and importance of colostrum are mentioned in Table 1.1.

Mature Milk

It is the breast milk that is produced after a few days. The quantity becomes larger, and the breasts feel full and heavy.

Property	*Importance*
Antibody-rich	Protects against infection and allergy
Many white cells	Protects against infection
Purgative	Clears meconium and helps prevent jaundice
Growth factors	Help intestine to mature
Vitamin A-rich	Reduces severity of infection, prevents eye disease

Table 1.1: Properties and importance of colostrum

Some people call this the breast milk "coming in".

Foremilk

Foremilk is the milk that is produced early in a feed. It looks bluer than hindmilk. It is produced in larger amounts and it provides plenty of water, proteins, lactose and other nutrients (Fig. 1.3A). Because a baby gets large amount of foremilk, she/he gets all the water that she/he needs from it. Babies do not need other drinks of water before they are 6 months old, even in a hot climate. God has given enough water and food in breast milk. Unnecessary interference by family members causes problems.

Hindmilk

Hindmilk is the milk that is produced later in a feed. It looks whiter than foremilk, because it contains more fat (Fig. 1.3B). This fat provides much of the energy of breastfed. This is an important reason not to take a baby off a breast too quickly. He should be allowed to continue until he has had all that she/he wants.

Two 25 ml samples of human breast milk pumped from the same woman, at the same time to illustrate what human breast milk looks like, and how human breast milk can vary. The left hand sample is foremilk, the first milk coming from a full breast. Foremilk has a higher water content and a lower fat content to satisfy thirst. The right hand sample is hindmilk, the last milk coming from a nearly empty breast. Hindmilk has a

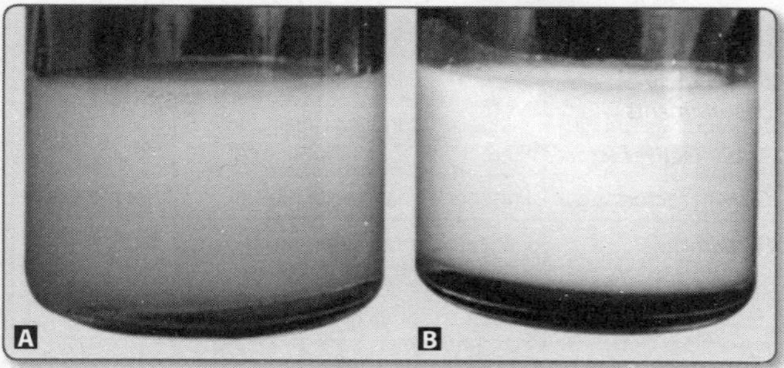

Figs 1.3A and B: (A) Foremilk; (B) Hindmilk

lower water content and a higher fat content to satisfy hunger. As breast milk is made continuously including during the feed itself, the milk can switch between foremilk and hindmilk until the baby has had enough. Switch on to second breast when first is completely empty.

Mechanisms of Protection against Infection

- When mother is infected
- White cells in mother's body make antibodies to protect her
- Some white cells go to her breast and make antibodies there
- These antibodies are secreted in breast milk to protect the baby.

Differences between Human Milk and Animal Milk

The differences between human milk and animal milk have been shown in Table 1.2 (Fig. 1.4).

Dangers of Artificial Feeding and Bottle Feeding

- More diarrhea, *acute respiratory infection* (ARI) and other infections
- Requires preparation
- Not easy to digest

	Human milk	*Animal milk*	*Formula*
Bacterial containments	None	Likely	Likely when mixed
Anti-infective factors	Present	Not present	Not present
Growth factors	Present	Not present	Not present
Protein	Correct amount easy to digest	Too much difficult to digest	Partly corrected
Fat	Enough essential fatty acids, lipase to digest	Lacks essential fatty acids, no lipase	Lacks essential fatty acids, no lipase
Iron	Small amount well absorbed	Small amount not well absorbed	Extra-added, not well absorbed
Vitamins	Enough	Not enough vitamin A and C	Vitamins added
Water	Enough	Extra-needed	May need extra

Table 1.2: Differences between human milk and animal milk

- Lacks balance of nutrients
- More likely to die from infection and malnutrition
- Increased risk of osteoporosis, ovarian and breast cancer

God has not made cow's and buffalo's
milk for human babies
Art by: Dr. Anil Mokashi
Built by: Swati Temkar. BPNI Maharashtra

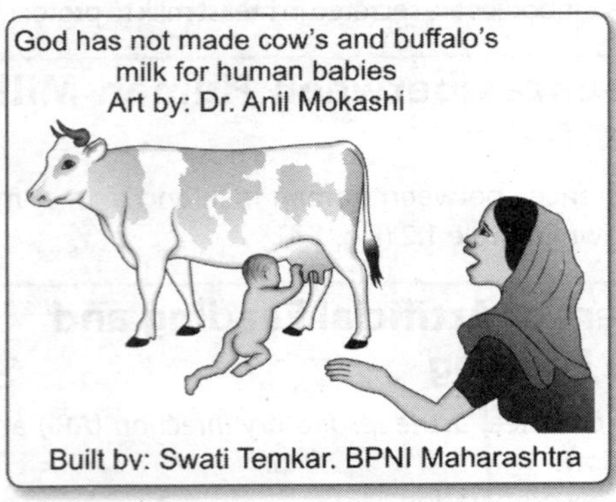

Fig. 1.4: Not made for each other

- Interferes with bonding
- More allergy and milk intolerance
- Increased risk of some chronic diseases
- Overweight babies
- Lower scores on intelligence tests
- Increased risk of anemia.

Recommendations

- Start breastfeeding within 1 hour of birth, no prelacteal feeds
- Practice exclusive breastfeeding from birth to 6 months of age
- Introduce appropriate complementary feeding after 6 months of age
- Sustain breastfeeding for 3 years and beyond
- Counsel HIV positive mothers to choose infant feeding option more suitable to them and support their decision
- Integrate infant and young child feeding with other health and nutrition services.

chapter 2

Production and Intake of Breast Milk

Introduction

You should know the anatomy and physiology of breastfeeding. If you understand how breastfeeding works, you will be able to help others.

Anatomy of the Breast

Amount of milk production does not depend on size of the breast. Large breast does not produce more milk. Small breast does not produce less milk. Breast size depends on fat and supporting tissue. Milk producing, storing and ejecting structures are not size dependent (Fig. 2.1).

Breasts contain:

- Milk secreting cells are called as alveoli. The hormone prolactin makes alveoli secrete milk
- Muscle cells are surrounding the alveoli. The hormone oxytocin makes them contract

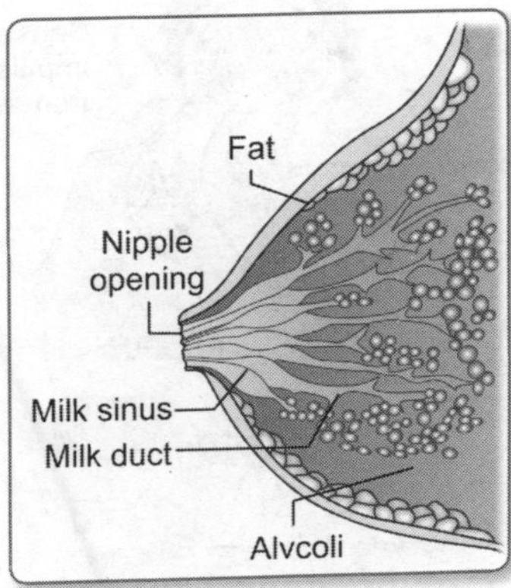

Fig. 2.1: Anatomy of the breast

- The ducts conduct the milk from alveoli to lactiferous sinuses. Ducts are situated in the breast below the areola
- Lactiferous sinuses are milk collecting cisterns. They are in the areola
- Nipple is only the "outlet" for milk.

Milk Production: the Prolactin Reflex

The prolactin reflex secreted after feed to produce next feed (Fig. 2.2).

Signs and Sensations of an Active Oxytocin Reflex

A mother may notice:

- A squeezing or tingling sensation in her breasts just before she feeds her baby or during a feed
- Milk flowing from her breasts when she thinks of her baby or hears his/her crying
- Milk dripping from her other breast, when her baby is sucking
- Milk flowing from her breasts in fine streams, if her baby comes off the breast during a feed

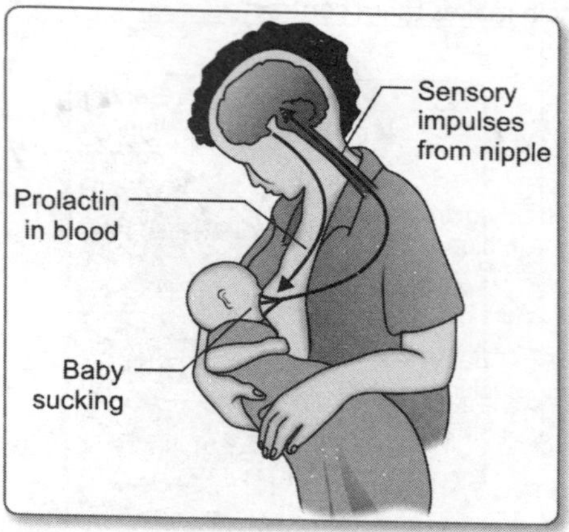

Fig. 2.2: Milk production: the prolactin reflex
Source: Adapted from WHO/UNICEF BFC, 1993.

- Pain from uterine contractions, sometimes with a rush of blood, during feeds in the first week
- Slow deep sucks and swallowing by the baby, which show that breast milk is flowing into his mouth.

Milk Flow: Oxytocin Reflex

The oxytocin reflex works before or during feed to make milk flow (Fig. 2.3).

Control of Breast Milk Production within the Breast

Sometimes mother complains that she gets milk from one breast. The other breast stops making milk. Actually the oxytocin and prolactin go equally to both breasts. Figures 2.2 and 2.3 shows why do these happen?

There is a substance in breast milk which can reduce or inhibit milk production. If a lot of milk is left in a breast, the inhibitor stops the cells from secreting any more. This helps to protect the breast from the harmful effects of being too full. It is obviously necessary if a baby dies or stops breastfeeding for some other reason. If breast milk is removed, by sucking or expression, the inhibitor is also removed. Then the breast

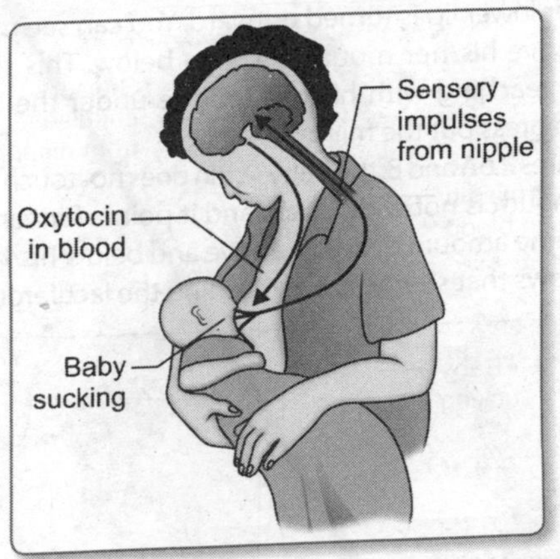

Fig. 2.3: Milk flow: the oxytocin reflex
Source: Adapted from WHO/UNICEF BFC, 1993

makes more milk. This helps you to understand why. If a baby stops suckling from one breast, that breast stops making milk. If a baby suckles more from one breast, that breast makes more milk and becomes larger than the other.

It also helps you to understand why. For a breast to continue to make milk, the milk must be removed. If a baby cannot suckle from one or both breasts or mother is not able to breastfeed, the breast milk must be removed by expression to enable production to continue.

Attachment at Breast—Inside the Mouth Appearance

Figures 2.4A and B show the same two babies attached to a breast.

The most important differences to see in Figures 2.4A and B are only the nipples which are in the mouth of babies, not the underlying breast tissue. The lactiferous sinuses are outside the baby's mouth, where his/her tongue cannot reach them. The baby's tongue is back inside his/her mouth, and not pressing on the lactiferous sinuses.

Attachment at Breast—Outside the Mouth Appearance

In Figures 2.5A and B, the baby's chin touches the breast. His/her mouth is wide open.

His/her lower lip is turned outward. You can see more of the areola above his/her mouth and less below. This shows that she/he is reaching with his/her tongue under the lactiferous sinuses to press out the milk.

In Figures 2.6A and B, the baby's chin does not touch the breast. His/her mouth is not wide open, and it points forward. You can see the same amount of areola above and below his/her mouth, which shows that she/he is not reaching the lactiferous sinuses.

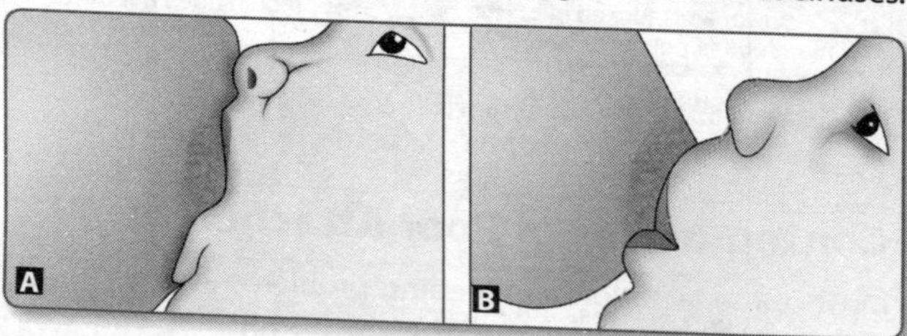

Figs 2.4A and B: (A) Well-attached baby; (B) Poorly-attached baby

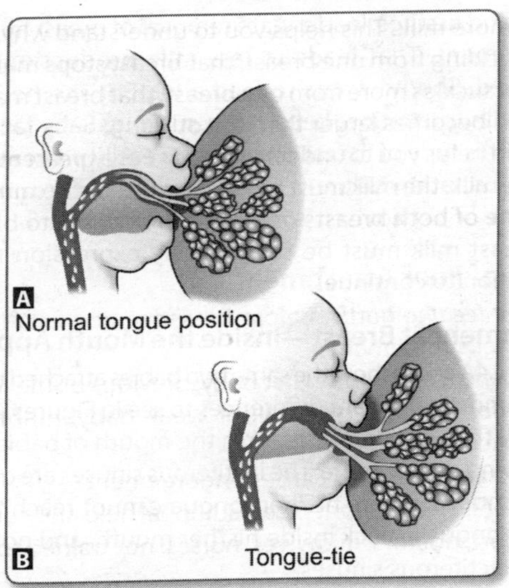

Figs 2.5A and B: Infant tongue position: (A) normal tongue position; (B) tongue-tie

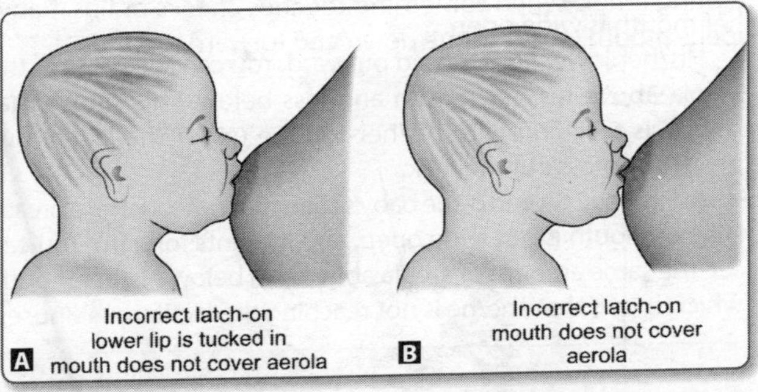

Figs 2.6A and B: Latch on: (A) incorrect latch on—lower lip is tucked in mouth does not cover aerola; (B) incorrect latch on—mouth does not cover aerola

Consequences of Poor Attachemnt

Most of the lactation and feeding problems are due to poor attachment. Pain and damage to the nipples cause sore nipples and fissures. Inadequate removal of breast milk causes engorgement. That leads to less milk production. Baby is unsatisfied. She/he wants to feed a lot. But she/he does not get milk. In frustration, baby stops sucking. Baby fails to gain weight. This type of "lactation failure" is easily preventable and curable. Lactation failure is never a failure of the mother, it is the failure of her adviser.

Causes of Poor Attachment

- *Use of feeding bottle:* Before breastfeeding established or for later supplements.
- *Inexperienced mother:* First baby, previous bottle feeder.
- *Functional difficulty:* Small or weak baby, nipple poorly protractile.
- Late starting to feed causes engorgement.
- *Lack of skilled support:* Less traditional help and community support, doctors, midwives, nurses, not trained to help.

Feeding Reflexes in Baby

Feeding reflexes in baby have been shown in Figure 2.7.

Rooting reflex: When something touches cheeks or lips, baby opens mouth, puts tongue down and forward.

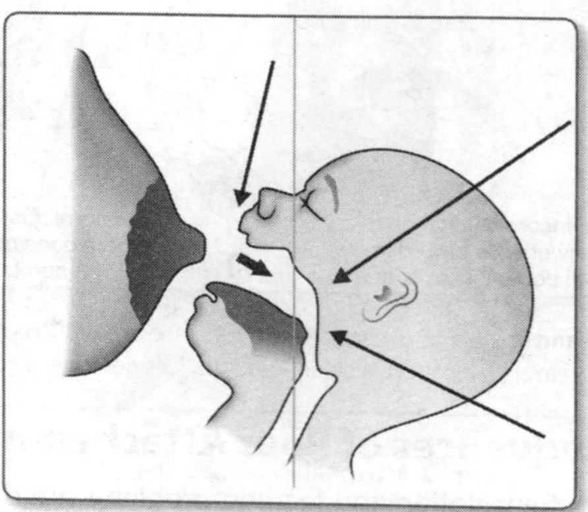

Fig. 2.7: Feeding reflexes in baby

Sucking reflex: When something touches palate baby sucks.

Swallowing reflex: When mouth fills with milk, baby swallows.

Summary

Breast milk flow depends partly on the mother's thoughts, emotions and sensations. It is important to keep mothers and babies together day and night, and to help mothers to feel good about breastfeeding. Many common difficulties can be caused by poor attachment to the breast. These difficulties can be overcome by helping a mother to correct her baby's position. They can be prevented by helping a mother to position her baby in the first few days.

The amount of milk that the breasts produce depends partly on how much the baby suckles, and how much milk she/he removes. More suckling makes more milk.

Most mothers can produce more milk than their babies can take, and they can produce enough for twins also.

Breastfeeding will be successful in most cases if:

- The mother feels good about herself
- The baby is well-attached to the breast so that she/he suckles effectively

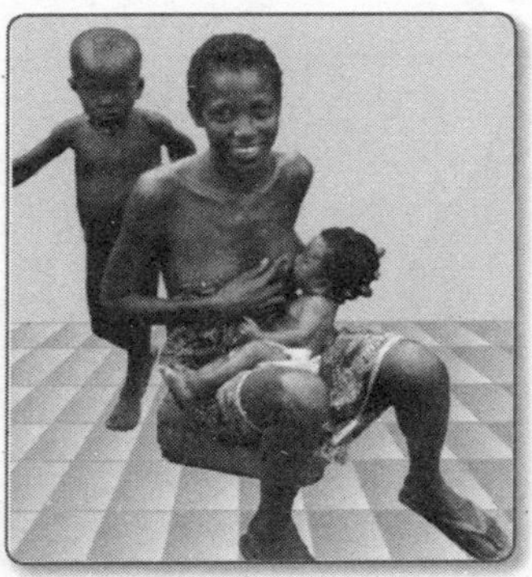

Fig. 2.8: A malnourished mother breastfeeds
Source: Adapted from Sierra Leone, 2001

- The baby suckles as often and for as long as she/he wants
- The environment supports breastfeeding.

Feed the mother and let her feed the infant. Monitor the weight and urine output. Temporary supplements by cup may be needed while the mother's milk production increases (Fig. 2.8) (© Joyce Kelly (ENN) 2001).

chapter 3

Assessing and Observing a Breastfeed

Introduction

Assessing a breastfeed helps you decide if a mother needs help or not, and how to help her. You can learn a lot about how well or bad breastfeeding is going by observing, before you ask questions. This is just as important part of clinical practice as other kinds of examination, such as looking for signs of dehydration, or counting how fast a child is breathing (Fig. 3.1).

How to Assess a Breastfeed?

- What do you notice about the mother?
- How does the mother hold her baby?
- What do you notice about the baby?
- How does the baby respond?
- How does the mother put her baby onto her breast?
- How does the mother hold her breast during a feed?
- Does the baby look well-attached to the breast?
- Is the baby suckling effectively?
- How does the breastfeed finish?
- Does the baby seem satisfied?

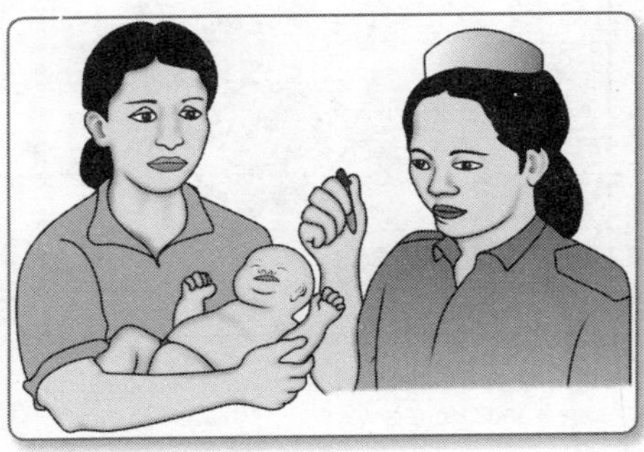

Fig. 3.1: Observing a breastfeed

- What is the condition of the mother's breasts?
- How does the mother feel when she is breastfeeding?

How Does the Mother Hold Her Baby While Breastfeeding (Fig. 3.2)?

Correct position: Baby's body close, facing breast. Face to face attention from mother.

Incorrect position: Baby's body away from mother. Baby's neck twisted. No mother baby eye contact.

How Does the Mother Hold Her Breast?

Correct holding: Resting her fingers on her chest wall. Her first finger forms a support at the base of the breast.

Incorrect holding: Holding her breast to close the nipple.

Breastfeed Obseravation Form

Mother's Name:

Date:

Baby's Name:

Age of Baby:

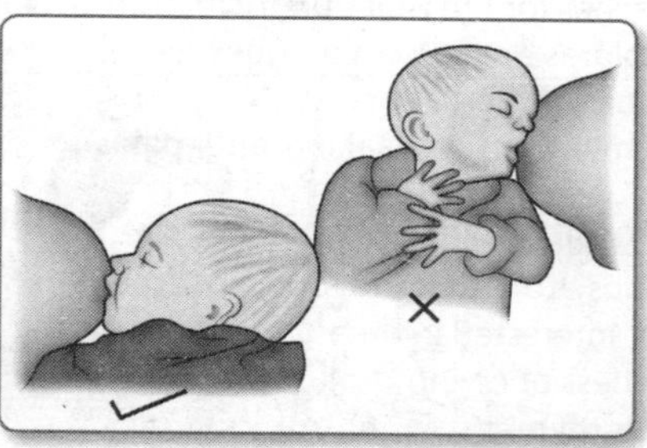

Fig. 3.2: Mother holds her baby while breastfeeding correct and incorrect ways

Body Position

Signs that Breastfeeding is Going Well

- Mother relaxed and comfortable
- Baby's head and body in straight line
- Baby's face facing breast
- Baby's nose opposite the nipple
- Baby's body close to mother's (baby's bottom supported)
- Baby reaches breast from below
- Breast well supported (optional)

Signs of Possible Difficulty

- Shoulders tense, leans over baby
- Baby's head and body is not in a straight line
- Baby's face not facing breast
- Baby's nose away from nipple
- Baby's body not close to mother
- Baby reached breast from above
- Breast supported in scissors hold or nipple being pushed in babies mouth

Response

Signs that Breastfeeding is Going Well

- Baby reaches for breast if hungry (baby roots for breast)
- Baby explores breast with tongue
- Baby calm and alert at breast
- Signs of milk ejection (leaking, after pains)

Signs of Possible Difficulty

- No response to breast (no rooting observed)
- Baby not interested in breast
- Baby restless or crying
- Baby slips off breast
- No signs of milk ejection

Emotional Bonding

Signs that Breastfeeding is Going Well

- Secure, confident hold
- Face-to-face attention from mother
- Much touching by mother

Signs of Possible Difficulty

- No response to breast (no rooting observed)
- Baby not interested in breast
- Baby restless or crying
- Baby slips off breast
- No signs of milk ejection

Anatomy

Signs that Breastfeeding is Going Well

- Breasts soft after feed
- Nipples average size
- Nipples stand out, protractile
- Skin appears healthy
- No lump in breast
- Breast looks round during feed

Signs of Possible Difficulty

- Breasts engorged
- Nipples large/flat/inverted
- Nipples not protractile
- Fissures or redness of skin
- Lump in breast
- Breast looks stretched or pulled

Suckling

Signs that Breastfeeding is Going Well

- Mouth wide open
- Chin touching the breast and nose close to breast
- Lower lip turned outward

- Tongue cupped around breast
- Cheeks round
- More areola above baby's mouth
- Slow deep sucks
- Can see or hear swallowing

Signs of Possible Difficulty

- Mouth not wide open, points forward
- Chin and nose away from the breast
- Lower lip turned in
- Baby's tongue not seen
- Cheeks tense or pulled in
- More areola below baby's mouth
- Rapid sucks only
- Can hear smacking or clicking

Time Spent Suckling

Sign that Breastfeeding is Going Well

- Baby releases breast

Sign of Possible Difficulty

- Mother takes baby off breast

Breastfeeding in all respects is best for both baby as well as for mother (Fig. 3.3).

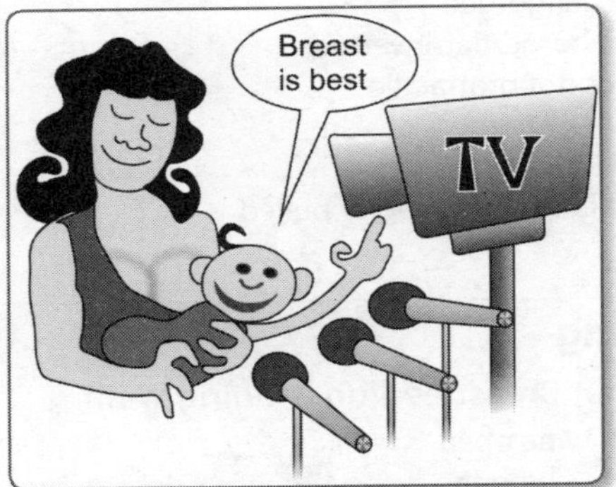

Fig. 3.3: Media can change the behavior

chapter

4

Feeding History

Introduction

If a mother asks for your help, you need to understand her situation. You cannot learn everything that you need to know by observing and listening and learning. You need to ask some questions.

Examples:

1. When the baby was born?
2. What happened at the time of delivery?
3. What else she feeds her baby?

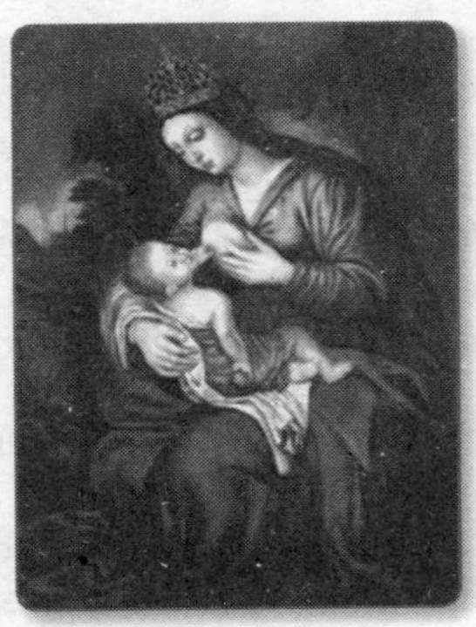

Fig. 4.1: Breastfeeding

How to Take a Feeding History?

Use the Mother's Name and the Baby's Name (If Appropriate)

Greet the women in a kind and friendly way. Introduce yourself, and ask her name and the baby's name. Remember and use them, or address her in whatever way is culturally appropriate.

Ask Her to Tell You about Herself and Her Baby in Her Own Way

Let her tell you first what she feels is important. You can learn the other things that you need to know later. Use your listening and learning skills to encourage her to tell you more.

Look at the Child's Growth Chart (Indian Growth Charts)

It may tell you some important facts and save you asking some questions.

Ask the Questions that will Tell You the Most Important Facts

You will need to ask questions, including some closed questions, but try not to ask too many. The breastfeeding History Form and Dietary Recall Form are guide to the facts that you may need to learn about. Decide what you need to know from each section of the two forms. In dietary recall form the caregiver is asked to recall everything the child consumed the previous day (foods, snacks, drinks, breastfeeds vitamin and mineral supplements). If the child is ill and did not eat his normal diet the previous day, ask the caregiver what the child eats on his normal eating day. Fill out the form with the answers.

Be Careful Not to Sound Critical

Ask questions politely. For example: Do not ask "Why are you bottle feeding?" It is better to say "What made you decide to give her some bottle feeds?" Use your confidence and support skills. Accept what the mother says, and praise what she is doing well.

Take Time to Learn about More Difficult, Sensitive Things

Some things are more difficult to ask about, but they can tell you about a woman's feelings, and whether she really wants to breastfeed. What have people told her about breastfeeding? Does she have to follow any special rules? What does the baby's father, mother or in-laws say? Did she want this pregnancy at this time? Is she happy about having the baby now? About the baby's sex? Some mothers tell you these things spontaneously. Others tell you when you empathize, and show that you understand how they feel. Others take longer. If a mother does not talk easily, wait and ask again later, or on another day, perhaps somewhere more private.

chapter 5

Listen What She Says, Tell What She Needs

Introduction

In "counseling" you understand how people feel, and help them to decide what to do. Here you will discuss with mother who are breastfeeding and how they feel. Most important counseling skills are "listening and learning" (Fig. 5.1).

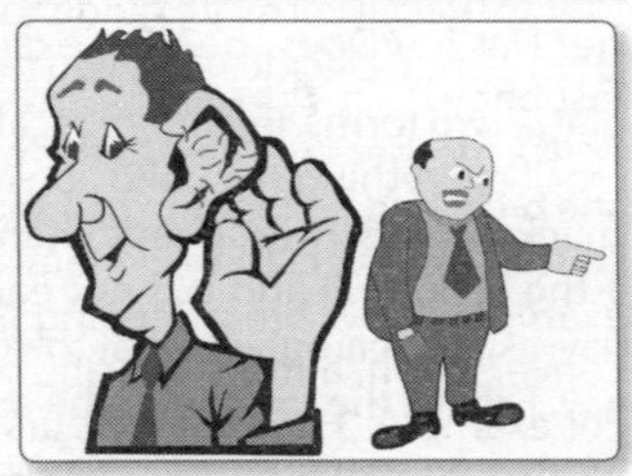

Fig. 5.1: Listening and learning are two important components of counseling

A breastfeeding mother may not talk about her feelings easily, especially if she is shy and with someone whom she does not know well. You need the skill to listen, and to make her feel that you are interested in her. This will encourage her to tell you more. She will be less likely to turn off, and say nothing.

Basic Counseling Skills

Skill 1: Use Helpful Nonverbal Communication

Nonverbal communication means showing your attitude through your posture, your expression, everything except through speaking. Helpful nonverbal communication makes a mother feel that you are interested in her, so it helps her to talk to you (Fig. 5.2).

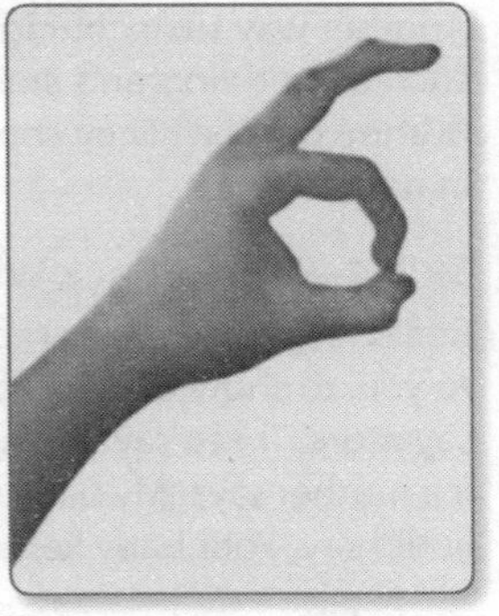

Fig. 5.2: Beautiful. You are right

Skill 2: Ask Open Questions

Open questions are very helpful. To answer them a mother must give you some information. Open questions usually start with

"How? What? When? Where? Why?" For example, "How are you feeding your baby?"

Closed questions are usually less helpful. They tell a mother the answer that you expect, and she can answer them with a "Yes" or "No". They usually start with words like "Are you? Did he? Has he? Does she?" For example, "Did you breastfeed your last baby?"

If a mother says "Yes" to this question, you still do not know if she breastfed exclusively, or if she also gave some artificial feeds. To start a conversation, general open questions are helpful. For example, "How breastfeeding is going for you? To continue a conversation, a more specific open question may be helpful. For example, "How many hours after he was born did he have his first feed?" Sometimes it is helpful to ask a closed question, make sure about a fact.

For example, "Are you giving him any other food or drink?" If she says "Yes", you can follow-up with an open question, to learn more. For example, "What made you decide to do that?" or "What are you giving him/her?"

Skill 3: Use Responses and Gestures Which Show Interest

Another way to encourage a mother to talk is to use gestures such as nodding and smiling, and simple responses such as "Mmm" or "Aha". They show a mother that you are interested in her.

Skill 4: Reflect Back What the Mother Says

Reflecting back means repeating back what a mother has said to you, to show that you have heard, and to encourage her to say more. Try to say it in a slightly different way. For example, if a mother says "My baby was crying too much last night". You could say "Your baby kept you awake crying all night".

Skill 5: Empathize—Show that You Understand How She Feels

Empathizing means showing that you understand how a person feels. For example, if a mother says "My baby wants to feed very often and it makes me feel so tired", you could say

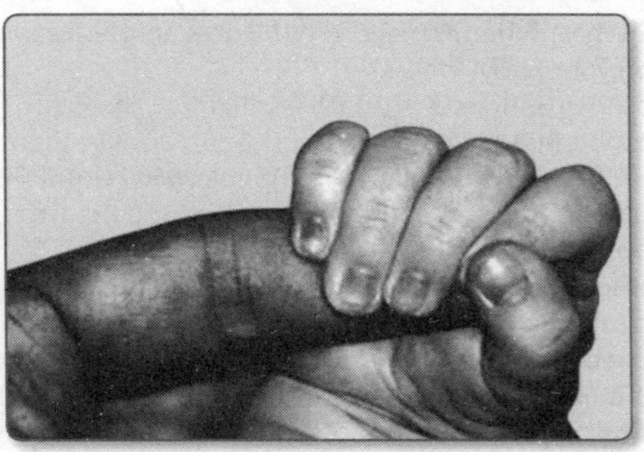

Fig. 5.3: Support

"You are feeling very tired all the time then". This shows that you understand that she feels tired, so you are empathizing. If you respond with a factual question, for example, "How often is she/he feeding? What else do you give him/her?" You are not empathizing (Fig. 5.3).

Skill 6: Avoid Words Which Sound Judging

Judging words are words like: right, wrong, well, badly, good, enough, properly. If you use these words when you ask questions, you may make a mother feel that she is wrong, or that there is something wrong with her baby. However, sometimes you need to use the "good" judging words to build a mother's confidence.

Listening and Learning Exercises

Asking Open Questions

Recognize the questions open or closed.

"Open question" which requires the mother to tell you more:

1. When was the last time you breastfed your baby?
2. How do you feed your baby now?

   So the above questions are open questions.

"Closed questions" can be answered "Yes" or "No":

1. Does your baby sleep with you?
2. Are you often away from your baby?
3. Are your nipples sore?

   So all the above three questions are closed questions.

Reflecting Back What a Mother Says

1. Mother says
   I do not have enough milk.
   You reflect back
   You think you do not have enough milk.
2. Mother says
   My baby is passing a lot of stools—sometimes 8 in a day.
   You reflect back
   He is passing many stools each day.
3. Mother says
   He doesn't seem to want to suckle from me.
   You reflect back
   He seems to be refusing to suckle.
4. Mother says
   I tried feeding him from a bottle, but he spat it out.
   You reflect back
   He refused to suck from a bottle.

Empathizing

Empathizing shows that you understand how she feels:

1. Mother says
   My baby wants to feed so often at night that I feel exhausted.
   You say
   You are really tired with the night feeding.
2. Mother says
   My nipples are so painful, I will stop breastfeeding.
   You say
   The pain makes you want to stop breastfeeding.
3. Mother says
   My breast milk looks so thin, I am sure it cannot be good.
   You say
   You are worried about how your breast milk looks.

4. Mother says
   I do not have any milk in my breasts, and my baby is a day old already.
   You say
   You are upset because your breast milk has not come in yet.
5. Mother says
   My breasts leak milk all day at work which is so embarrassing.
   You say
   I agree it must be embarrassing, especially when you are in your office. I would suggest you express out.

Judging Words

Judging words are: well, normal, enough, problem, crying, "too much" good, correct, adequate, fail, unhappy, bad, proper, inadequate, failure, happy, badly, right, satisfied, succeed fussy, wrong, plenty of, success, colicky, sufficient.

Judging Questions

- Does he suckle well?
- Are his stools normal?
- Is he gaining enough weight?
- Do you have any problem of breastfeeding?
- Does he cry too much at night?

In Clinical Practice

- Introduce yourself to the mother, and ask her permission to talk to her. Introduce if you are in a group, and explain that you are interested in infant feeding.
- Try to find a chair or stool to sit on.
- If the baby is feeding, ask the mother to continue as she is doing. If the baby is not feeding, ask the mother to give a feed in the normal way at any time that the baby seems ready: ask the mother's permission to watch the feed.
- Before or after the breastfeed, ask the mother some open questions. "How she is, how the baby is, and how feeding is going on" to start conversation. Encourage the mother

to talk about herself and the baby. Practice as many of the listening and learning skills as possible.

Mistakes to Avoid

- Do not say that you are interested in "breastfeeding". The mother's behavior may change. You should say that you are interested in "infant feeding" or in "how babies feed".
- Do not give a mother help or advice without her consent.

chapter 6

Baby-friendly Hospital

Introduction

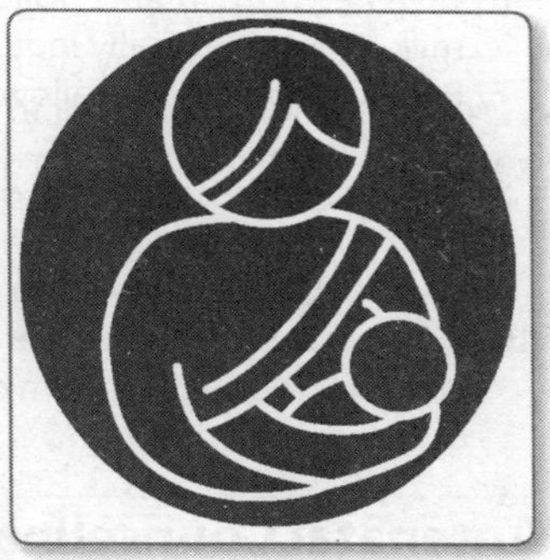

Fig. 6.1: Breastfeeding symbol

Hospital practices are important. They can improve or hamper the successful breastfeeding. Wrong practices can be effectively changed (Fig. 6.1). Change is always difficult. But you have to change for better. It is difficult to tell the hospital doctors and staff that they are doing wrong. But as a trained person, that is your job. And you have to do it skillfully. Poor hospital practices interfere with natural breastfeeding and contribute to the spread of artificial feeding.

Maternity homes should help mothers to:

- Start breastfeeding at the time of delivery
- Establish breastfeeding in the postnatal period
- Sustain breastfeeding up to 2 years or beyond
- Timely introduction of complementary feeding
- Skin to skin contact in the first hour after delivery helps breastfeeding and bonding.

Ten Steps to Successful Breastfeeding

Every maternity home should:

1. Have a written breastfeeding policy that is routinely communicated to all health care staff
2. Train all health care staff in skills necessary to implement this policy
3. Inform all pregnant women about the benefits and management of breastfeeding

4. Help mothers initiate breastfeeding within half an hour birth
5. Show mothers how to breastfeed, and how to maintain lactation even if they are separated from their infants
6. Give newborn infants no food or drink other than breast milk, unless medically indicated
7. Practice rooming-in—allow mothers and infants to remain together 24 hours a day
8. Encourage breastfeeding on demand
9. Give no artificial teats or pacifiers (also called dummies or soothers) to breastfeeding infants
10. Foster the establishment of breastfeeding support groups and refer mothers to them on discharge from the hospital or clinic.

Antenatal Counseling for Breastfeeding

Antenatal counseling is a job of lactation management counselor. It gives you an opportunity to get introduced to the expecting mother so that she knows whom to approach in case she has any problems (Fig. 6.2).

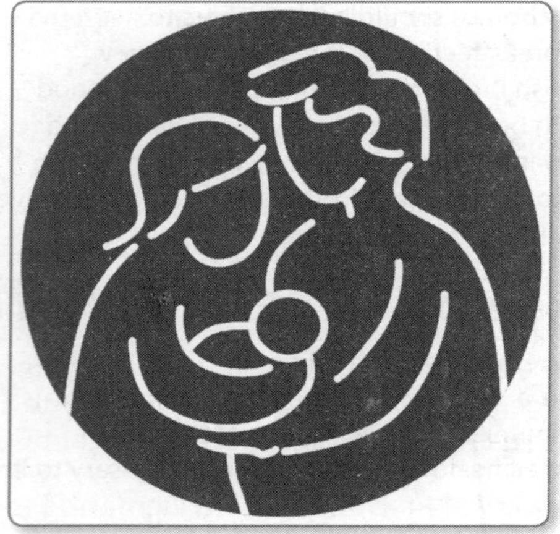

Fig. 6.2: Counseling service in hospitals

With Mothers in Groups

- Explain benefits of breastfeeding
- Give simple relevant information on how to breastfeed
- Explain what happens after delivery
- Discuss mother's questions.

With Each Mother Individually

- Ask about previous breastfeeding experience
- Ask if she has any questions or worries
- Examine her breasts only if she is worried about them
- Build her confidence and explain that you will help her.

Dangers of Prelacteal Feeds

Prelacteal feeds are artificial feeds of drinks given to a baby before breastfeeding is initiated.

They are dangerous because:

- They replace colostrum as the baby's earliest feeds
- The baby is more likely to develop infections, such as diarrhea, septicemia and meningitis
- He is more likely to develop intolerance to the proteins in the artificial feed, and allergies, such as eczema
- They interfere with suckling
- The baby's hunger is satisfied, and hence breastfeeds less
- If she/he is fed from a bottle with an artificial teat, she/he may have more difficulty attaching to the breast, (nipple confusion)
- The baby suckles and stimulates the breast less
- Breast milk takes longer to "come in" and it is more difficult to establish breastfeeding if a baby has even a few prelacteal feeds; Mother is more likely to have difficulties, such as engorgement. Breastfeeding is more likely to stop early when a baby is exclusively breastfed from birth.

Advantages of Rooming-in and Demand Feeding

Rooming-in (ideally bedding-in) and demand feeding help bonding and breastfeeding.

Advantages of rooming-in:
- Mother can respond to baby, which helps bonding
- Babies cry less, so less temptation to give bottle feeds
- Mothers more confident about breastfeeding
- Breastfeeding continues longer.

Advantages of demand feeding:
- Breast milk "comes in" sooner
- Baby gains weight faster
- Fewer difficulties such as engorgement
- Breastfeeding more easily established.

How to Help a Mother with an Early Breastfeed?

Avoid Hurry and Noise

Talk quietly, and be unhurried, even if you have only a few minutes to ask the mother how she feels and how breastfeeding is going. Let her tell you how she feels, before you give any information or suggestions.

Observe a Breastfeed

Try to see the mother when she is feeding her baby, and quietly watch what is happening. If the baby's position and attachment are good, tell her how well she and the baby are doing. You do not need to show her what to do (Fig. 6.3).

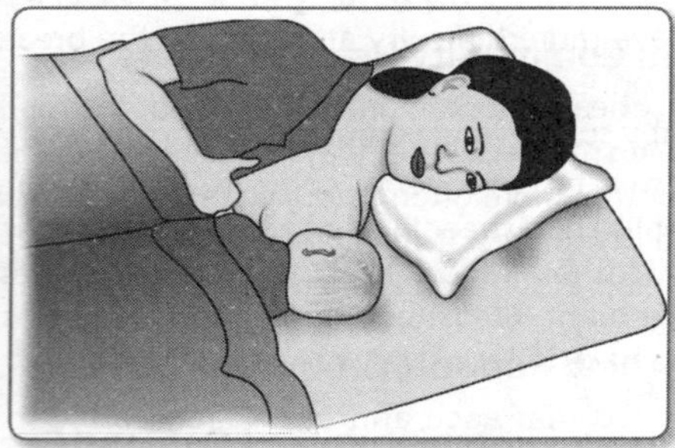

Fig. 6.3: Rooming-in

Help with Positioning If Necessary

If the mother is having difficulty, or if her baby is not well attached, give her appropriate help.

Give Her Relevant Information

Make sure that she understands about demand feeding, about the signs that a baby gives that show that he is ready to feed, and explain how her milk will "come in".

Answer the Mother's Questions

She may have some questions that she wants to ask. Explain simply and clearly what she needs to know.

Sources of Help for Breastfeeding Mothers

Supportive Family and Friends

This is often the most important source of support. Community success is often good where breastfeeding traditions are strong, and family members live near. Many women, especially in cities, have little support. Or they may have friends or relatives who encourage them to bottle feed.

Postnatal Check, within 1 Week and 6 Weeks

This check should include observation of a breastfeed, and discussion of how breastfeeding is going. You can help mothers with minor difficulties before they become serious problems.

Help from Community Health Workers

Community health workers are often in a good position to help breastfeeding mother, as they may live nearby. They may be able to see a mother more often, and give more time, than facility-based health workers. It may be helpful to train community health workers in some breastfeeding counseling skills.

Breastfeeding Support Group

It is expected that each and every lactation management counselor promotes a local mother support group (MSG) and acts as a leader (Fig. 6.4).

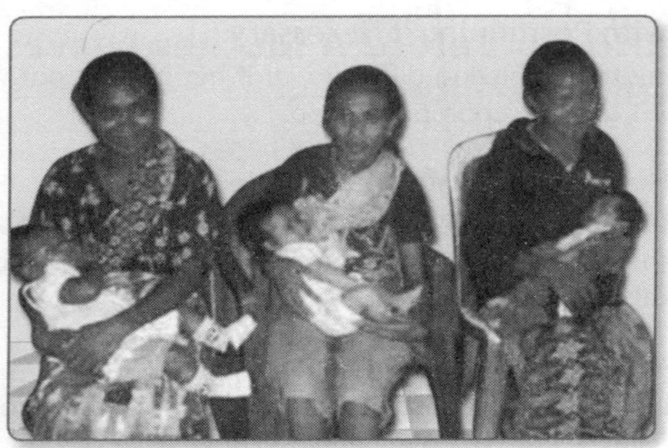

Fig. 6.4: Local mother support group

A group may be started by a lactation management counselor (LMC); by an existing women's group; by a group of mothers who feel that breastfeeding is important; or by mothers who meet and help each other

A group of breastfeeding mothers meets together every 1–4 weeks, often in one of their homes, or somewhere in the community. They can have a topic to discuss, such as "The advantages of breastfeeding" or "Overcoming difficulties"

They share experiences, and help each other with encouragement and with practical ideas about how to overcome difficulties. They learn more about how their bodies work

The group needs someone who is accurately informed about breastfeeding to train them. They need someone who can correct any mistaken ideas, and suggest solutions to difficulties. This helps the group to be positive

The group needs a source of information whom they can refer to if they need help. This could be health worker trained in breastfeeding, whom they see from time to time. The group also needs up-to-date materials to educate themselves about breastfeeding

Mothers can also help each other at other times, and not only at meeting. They can visit each other when they are worried or depressed, or when they do not know what to do.

What to Do Before A Mother Leaves A Maternity Facility?

- Find out what support she has at home
- If possible, talk to family members about her needs
- Arrange a postnatal check in the first week, which includes observation of a breastfeed (in addition to a routine check at 6 weeks)
- Make sure that she knows how to contact a health worker who can help with breastfeeding if necessary
- If there is a breastfeeding support group in her neighborhood, refer her to that.

chapter 7

Positioning a Baby at the Breast

Introduction

Always observe mother breastfeeding before you help her. See what she is doing. Try to understand her situation clearly. Do not rush to make her do something different (Fig. 7.1).

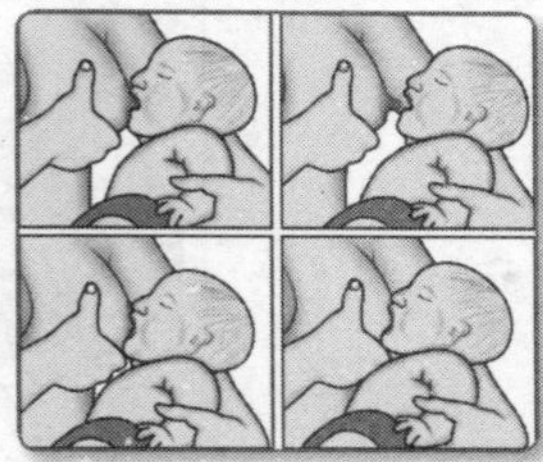

Fig. 7.1: Baby positioning

Give A Mother Help Only If She has Difficulty

Some mothers breastfeed to their babies satisfactorily. There is no point in disturbing and teaching something new. Baby and mother should be comfortable. Let the mother do as much as possible herself. Do not "take over" from her. Explain what you want her to do. If possible, demonstrate to show her what you mean. See that she understands, so that she can do it herself. Your aim is to help her to position her own baby.

How to Help A Mother Who is Sitting?

- Make sure that she is sitting in a comfortable position (Fig. 7.2)
- Sit down yourself so that you also are comfortable and relaxed, and at a same level
- Explain to the mother how to hold her baby
  Make these four key points clear:
  - The baby's head and body should be in a straight line
  - Baby's face should face the breast, with nose opposite the nipple
  - Mother should hold the baby close to her with skin to skin contact
  - She should support his bottom, and not just his head and shoulders.

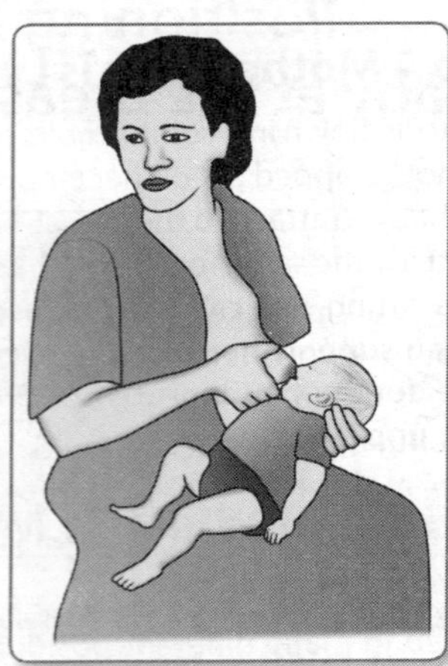

Fig. 7.2: A sitting mother breastfeeding her baby

- Show her how to support her breast with her "C" shaped or cupped hand
- She should rest her fingers on her chest wall under her breast so that her first finger forms a support at the base of the breast. She can use her thumb to press the top of her breast slightly. This can improve the shape of the breast so that it is easier for her baby to attach well. She should not hold her breast too near to the nipple
- Explain how she should touch her baby's lips with her nipple so that she/he opens his/her mouth
- Explain that she/he should wait until her/her baby's mouth is wide open before she moves him/her onto her/his breast. His/her mouth needs to be open to take a large mouthful of breast
- Explain or show her how to quickly move her baby to her breast when she/he is opening his/her mouth wide. She should bring her baby to her breast and not herself or her breast to the baby. She should aim her baby's lower lip below her nipple so that his/her tongue will touch her breast
- Lastly she/he should have an eye to eye contact with the baby while the baby is enjoying feeds.

How to Help A Mother Who is Lying Down?

Help the mother to lie down in a comfortable, relaxed position. It is better she is not "propped up" on her elbow. This can make it difficult for the baby to attach to the breast. Show her how to hold her baby. Exactly the same four key points are important, as for a mother is sitting, she can support her baby with her lower arm. She can support her breast if necessary with her upper arm. If she does not support her breast, she can hold her baby with her upper arm.

Other Positions in Which A Mother Can Breastfeed

Mothers breastfeed in many different positions, for example standing up. It is important for the mother to be comfortable and relaxed and for her baby to take enough of the breast into his mouth so that he can suckle effectively. Some useful positions that you may want to show mothers are:

- The underarm position (useful for twins, blocked duct, difficulty attaching the baby) (Fig. 7.3)

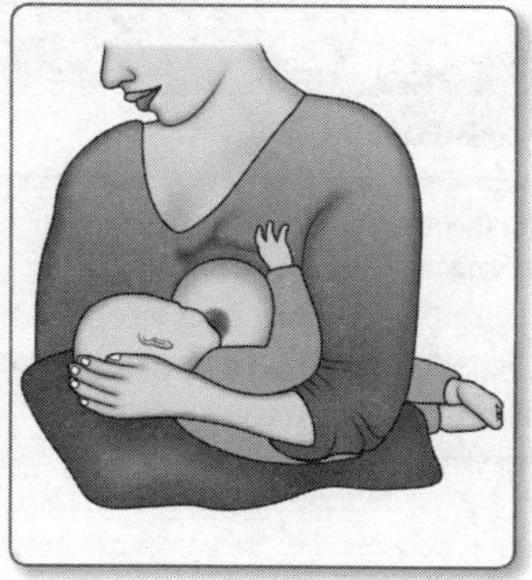

Fig. 7.3: A mother holding her baby in the underarm position (feeding position: football/clutch)

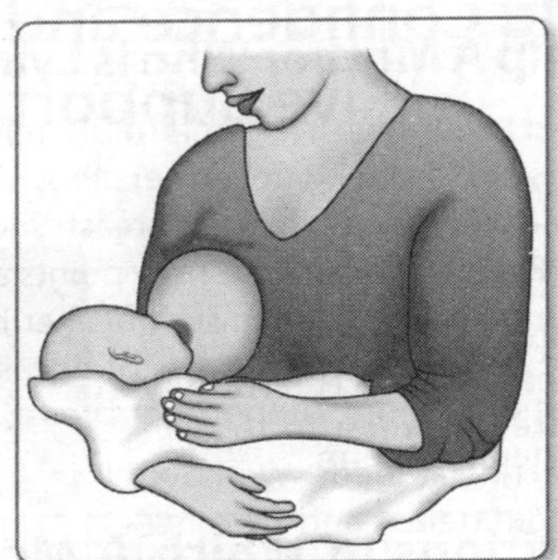

Fig. 7.4: A mother holding her baby with arm to the opposite breast (feeding position: cradle)

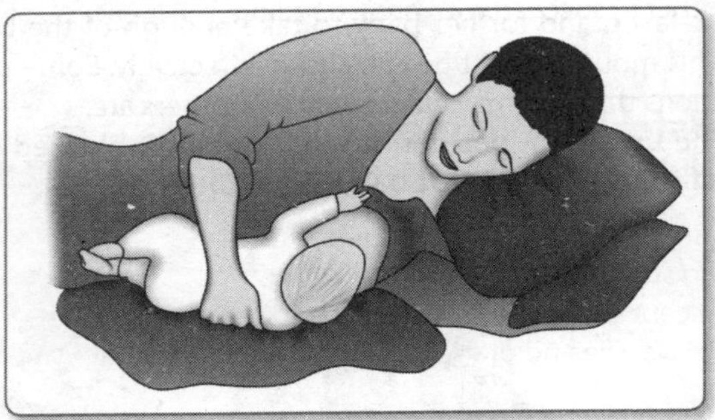

Fig. 7.5: A mother breastfeeding her baby lying down (feeding position: side-lying using modified cradle)

- Holding the baby with the arm opposite the breast (useful for very small babies, sick babies) (Fig. 7.4)
- Breastfeeding while lying down (Fig. 7.5).

chapter 8

Build Confidence and Give Support

Introduction

A breastfeeding mother easily loses confidence in herself. Her family and friends create pressure to give unnecessary artificial feeds. We have to build her confidence and give her support. Confidence helps her to resist pressures from other people. You need the skill to help her to feel confident and good about herself. Confidence can help a mother to succeed with breastfeeding (Fig. 8.1).

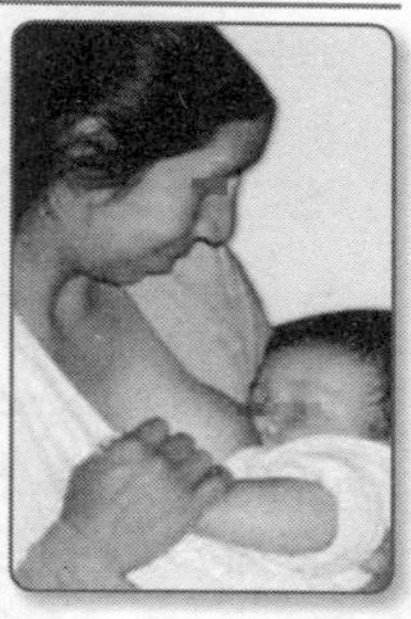

Fig. 8.1: A confident mother breastfeeding her baby
Source: Adapted from Guatemala/LINKAGES, Maryanne Stone-Jimenez.

Skills for Building Confidence and Giving Support

The skills for building confidence and giving support include the following:

- Accept what a mother thinks and feels
- Recognize and praise what the mother and baby are doing right
- Give practical help
- Give little relevant information and check understanding
- Use simple language
- Make one or two suggestions, not commands.

Skill 1: Accept What a Mother Thinks and Feels

Never say that she is wrong. This reduces her confidence. It is more helpful to accept what she thinks. Accepting means responding in a neutral way. Show your interest and acceptance. Sometimes a mother feels very upset about a minor thing. If you say "Do not worry, there is nothing to worry about!" She feels that you are not understanding her problem, and it

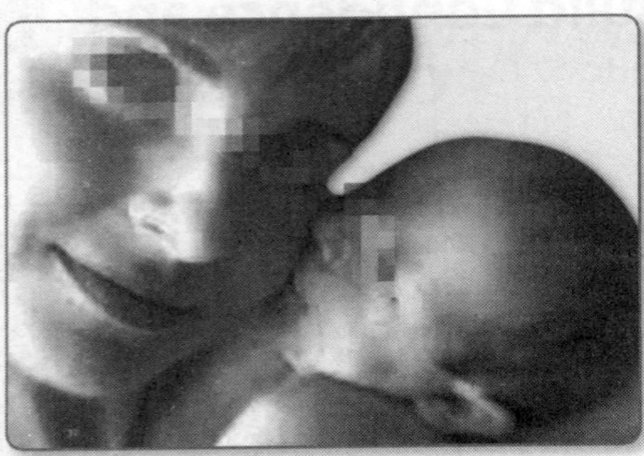

Fig. 8.2: Bonding

reduces her confidence. Reflecting back and empathizing with her feelings is useful (Fig. 8.2).

Skill 2: Recognize and Praise What the Mother and Baby are Doing Right

We try to look for "problems". We try to find "mistakes" and correct them. It is not a very good approach of solving problems. We should not try to be advisers. As counselors, we must learn to look for and recognize what mothers and babies do right. Then we should praise or show approval of the good practices. Praising good practices have these benefits:

- It builds a mother's confidence
- It encourages her to continue those good practices
- It makes it easier for her to accept suggestions later.

Skill 3: Give Little Relevant Information and Check Understanding

Tell her something that is important now. That she can do today. Only one or two things at a time. Accept what she says, praise what she her baby do right, build her confidence in you. Ask question to find out whether she has understood. Give further explanation if needed.

Skill 4: Use Simple Language

Use simple familiar terms to explain things to mothers. Avoid the technical terms.

Skill 5: Make One or Two Suggestions, Not Commands

Do not order, but suggest. If you give commands she loses confidence. Instead, suggest what she could do differently. Then she can decide if she will try it or not. This leaves her feeling in control, and helps her to feel confident.

chapter 9

Breast Problems

Introduction

Many breast conditions cause difficulties with breastfeeding. Diagnosis and management of these breast conditions are important both to relieve the mother and to enable breastfeeding to continue. These breast conditions are:

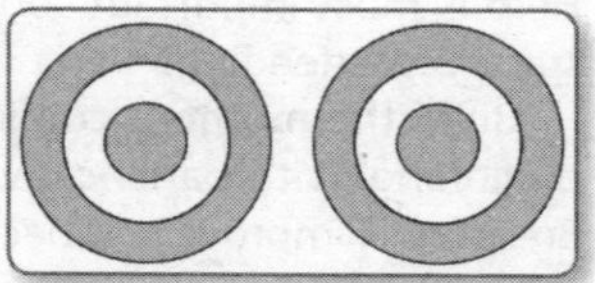

Fig. 9.1A: Breast problems are an emergency

- Flat or inverted nipples, and long or big nipples
- Engorgement
- Blocked duct and mastitis
- Sore nipples and nipple fissure.

There are many shapes and sizes of breast. Babies can successfully breastfeed from all "shapes and sizes" of breasts and nipples (Figs 9.1A and B).

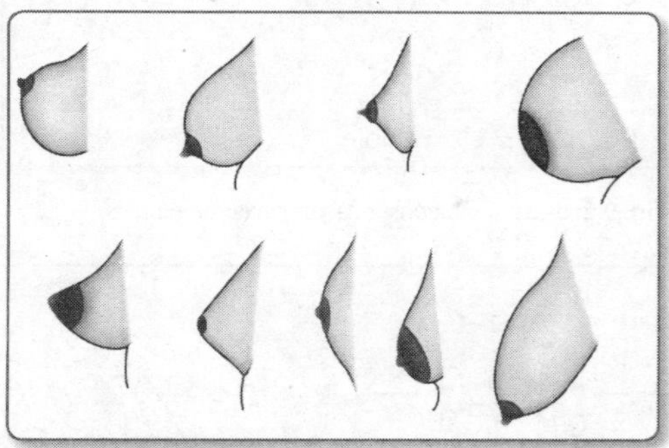

Fig. 9.1B: Different shapes and sizes of breasts

Management of Flat and Inverted Nipples (Figs 9.2 to 9.4)

Antenatal treatment is probably not helpful. For example, stretching nipples or wearing nipple shells does not help. Most nipples improve around the time of delivery without treatment. Help is most important soon after delivery, when the baby starts breastfeeding:

Build the mother's confidence. It may be difficult at the beginning. With patience and persistence she can succeed. Breasts will improve and become softer in a week or two after delivery. Baby's suckle will help to pull her nipples out. Baby suckles from the breast not the nipple. Baby needs to take a large mouthful of breast. As baby breastfeeds, she/he will pull the breast and nipple out.

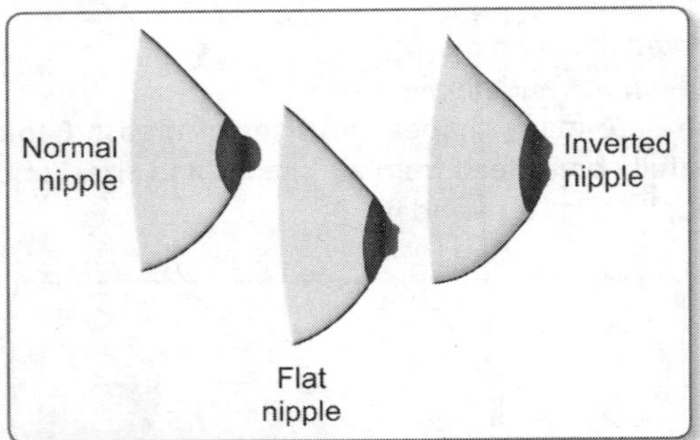

Fig. 9.2: Breast conditions—flat and inverted nipples

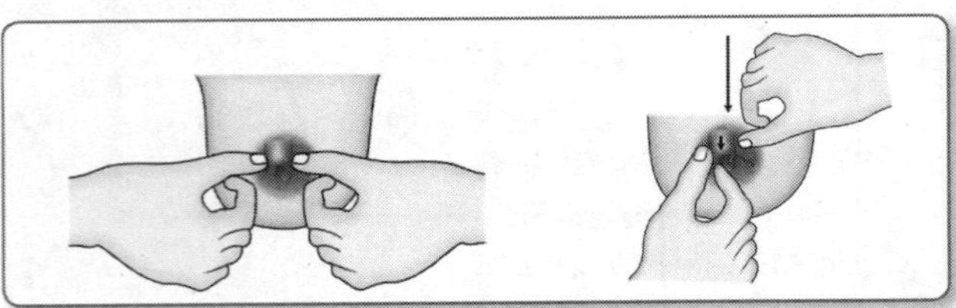

Fig. 9.3: How to treat flat, inverted nipple

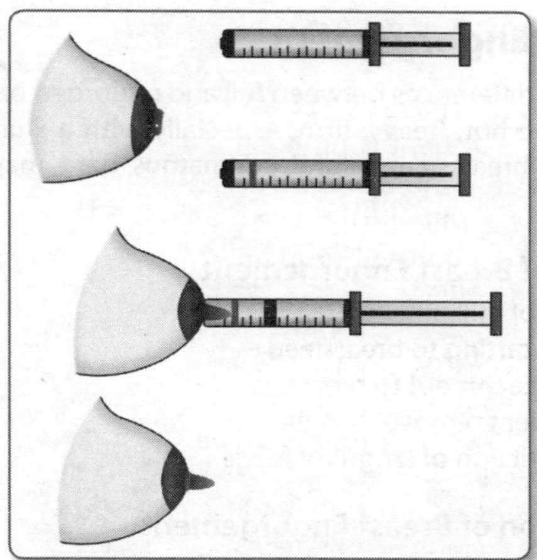

Fig. 9.4: Preparing and using a syringe for treatment of inverted nipples

Encourage her to give plenty of skin to skin contact. Help her to position her baby. Give her this help early, in the first day, before breast milk comes on, and her breasts are full. Help her to try different position to hold her baby.

If a baby cannot suckle effectively in the first week or two, help his mother to express her milk and feed it to her baby with a cup. Expressing milk helps to keep breasts soft so that it is easier for the baby to attach the breast; and it helps to keep up the supply of breast milk. She/he should not use a bottle because that makes it more difficult for her/his baby to take her/him breast.

Express a little milk directly into her baby's mouth. Some mothers find that this is helpful. The baby gets some milk straight away, so she/he is less frustrated. She/he may be more willing to try to suckle. Mother should continue to give him/her skin to skin contact.

Breast Engorgement

Know the differences between full and engorged breasts. Full breasts are hot, heavy, firm, especially with a shiny nipple. Engorged breasts are painful, edematous, hard, may look red (Fig. 9.5).

Causes of Breast Engorgement

- Plenty of milk
- Delay starting to breastfeed
- Poor attachment to breast
- Infrequent removal of milk
- By restriction of length of feeds.

Prevention of Breast Engorgement

- Start breastfeeding soon after delivery
- Ensure good attachment
- Encourage unrestricted breastfeeding.

Treatment of Breast Engorgement

To treat engorgement, it is essential to remove milk. If milk is not removed, mastitis may develop, an abscess may form and breast milk production decreases. So do not advise a mother "rest" the breast. If the baby is able to suckle, he/she should

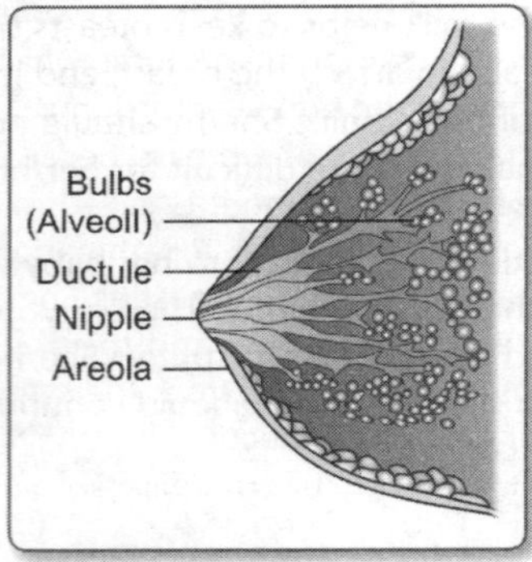

Fig. 9.5: Structure inside breast

feed frequently. This is the best way to remove milk. Help the mother to position her baby so that he/she attaches well. Then baby suckles effectively, and does not damage the nipple. If the baby is not able to suckle, help her to express milk. She may be able to express by hand or breast pump (Fig. 9.4), or a warm bottle. Expressing a little milk will make the breast soft enough for the baby to suckle. Before feeding or expressing, stimulate the mother's oxytocin reflex.

These are things that she can do:

- Put a warm compress on her breasts
- Massage her neck and back
- Massage her breast lightly
- Stimulate her breast and nipple skin
- Help her to relax.

After a feed, put a cold compress on her breasts. This may help to reduce edema. Build the mother's confidence. Explain that she will soon be able to breastfeed comfortably.

Blocked Duct and Mastitis

Mastitis may develop in an engorged breast, or it may follow a condition called blocked duct.

Symptoms of Blocked Duct and Mastitis

Blocked duct occurs when the milk is not removed from part of a breast. The duct to that part of the breast is sometimes blocked by thickened milk. The symptoms are lump which is tender, and sometimes redness of the skin over the lump.

When milk stays in part of a breast, because of a blocked duct, because of engorgement, it is called milk stasis. If the milk is not removed, it can cause inflammation of the breast tissue, which is called noninfective mastitis. Sometimes a breast becomes infected with bacteria, and this is called infective mastitis. It is not possible to tell from the symptoms alone if mastitis is noninfective or infective. If the symptoms are all severe; however, the woman is more likely to need treatment with antibiotics.

Causes of Blocked Duct and Mastitis

The main cause of blocked duct and mastitis is poor drainage of all or part of a breast. Infrequent breastfeeds is the main reason of poor drainage.

- When a mother is very busy
- When her baby starts feeding less often because she/he sleeps through the night, or feeds irregularly
- Because of a changed feeding pattern for any other reason, for example, a journey
- Ineffective suckling if the baby is poorly attached to the breast
- Pressure from tight clothes, usually a bra, especially if she wears it at night; or from lying on the breast, which can block one of the ducts
- Pressure of the mother's fingers, which can block milk flow during a breastfeed. The lower part of a large breast drains poorly, because of the way in which the breast hangs
- Another important factor is stress and overwork of the mother, probably because it causes her to breastfeed her baby less often, or for shorter times
- Trauma to the breast which damages breast tissue sometimes causes mastitis, for example, a sudden blow or an accidental kick by an older child
- If there is a nipple fissure, it provides a way for bacteria to enter the breast tissue. This is another way in which poor attachment can lead to mastitis.

Treatment of Blocked Duct and Mastitis

- Improve the drainage of milk from the affected part of the breast
- Look for a cause of poor drainage, and correct it
- Look for poor attachment
- Look for pressure from clothes, usually a tight bra, especially if worn at night; or pressure from lying on the breast
- Notice what the mother does with her fingers as she breastfeeds. Does she hold the areola, and possibly block milk flow?

- Notice if she has large, pendulous breasts, and if the blocked duct is in the lower part of her breast (if so, suggest that she lift the breast more while she feeds the baby, to help the lower part of the breast to drain better).

Sometimes advice the mother to do the following things:

- Breastfeed frequently
- Show her how to massage over the blocked area, and over the duct which leads from the blocked area, right down to the nipple. This helps to remove the milk from the duct. She may notice that a plug of thickened milk comes out with her milk (it is safe for the baby to swallow the plug)
- Apply warm compresses to her breast between feeds.

Sometimes it is helpful to do these things:

- Start the feed on the unaffected breast. This may help if pain seems to preventing the oxytocin reflex. Change to the affected breast after the reflex starts working.
- Breastfeed the baby in different positions at different feeds. This helps to remove milk from different parts of the breast more equally. Show the mother how to hold her baby in the underarm position, or how to lie down to feed him, instead of holding him across the front at every feed.

Additional Treatment

A mother needs additional treatment if there are:

- Severe symptoms when you first see her (Fig. 9.6)
- A fissure, through which bacteria can enter
- No improvement after 24 hours of improved drainage.

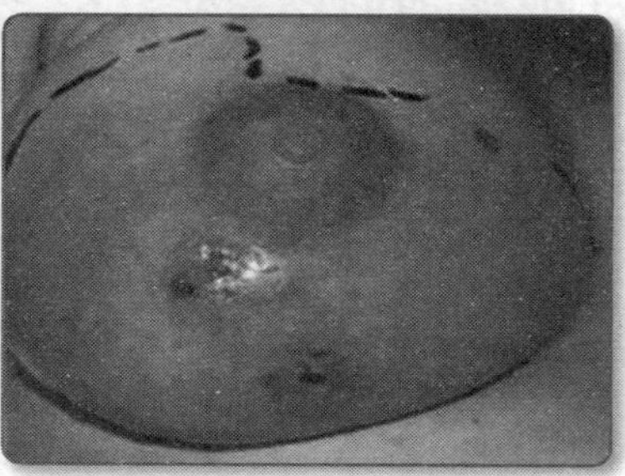

Fig. 9.6: Mastitis

Treat her, or refer her for treatment with the following:

Antibiotics: Amoxicillin or amoxyclavulanic acid combination—it is important to complete the dose of antibiotics as prescribed by the doctor. Complete rest. Advice her to take sick leave, if she is employed, or to get help at home with her duties.

Analgesics: Give her ibuprofen or paracetamol for the pain. Explain that she should continue with frequent breastfeeds, massage and warm compresses. If she is not eating well, encourage her to adequate food and fluids.

Treatment of Candida Infection (Figs 9.7A to C)

To baby mouth—apply fluconazole oral paint.
To mothers breast—apply fluconazole cream.

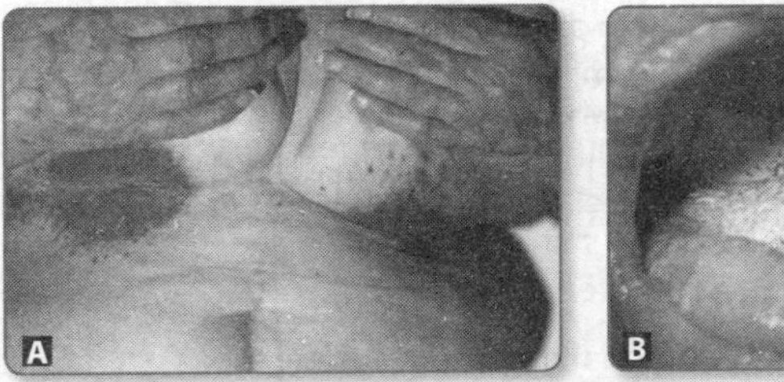

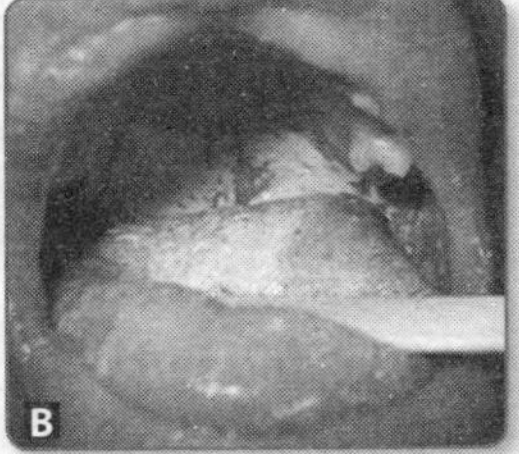

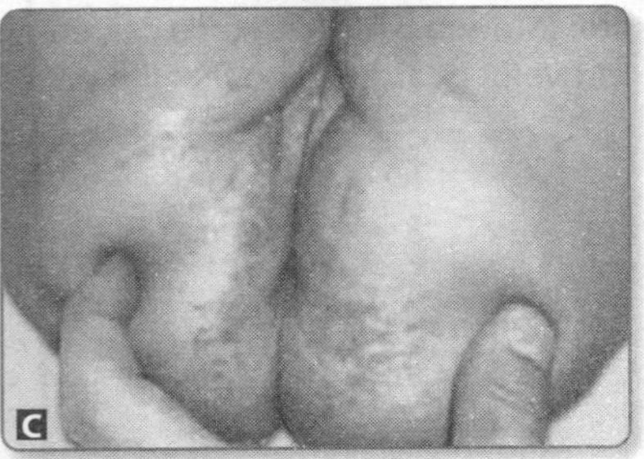

Figs 7A to C: Candidiasis: breast intertrigo, oral, perianal-pereneal

When either of them has candidial infections both should be treated to prevent "ping pong" infection. Stop using pacifiers, teats and nipple shields.

Management of Sore Nipples

First Look for a Cause

Observe the baby breastfeeding. Check for signs of poor attachment. Examine the breasts. Look for engorgement. Look for fissures. Look baby's mouth for signs of Candida and baby's bottom for Candida rash.

Give Appropriate Treatment

Build the mother's confidence. Explain that soreness is temporary, and that soon breastfeeding will be completely comfortable. Help her to improve her baby's attachment. Often this is all that is necessary. She can continue breastfeeding, and need not rest her breast. Help her to reduce engorgement if necessary. She should breastfeed frequently or express her breast milk. Consider treatment for Candida if the skin of the nipple and areola is red, shiny or flaky; or if there is itchiness, or deep pain, or if the soreness persists (Fig. 9.8).

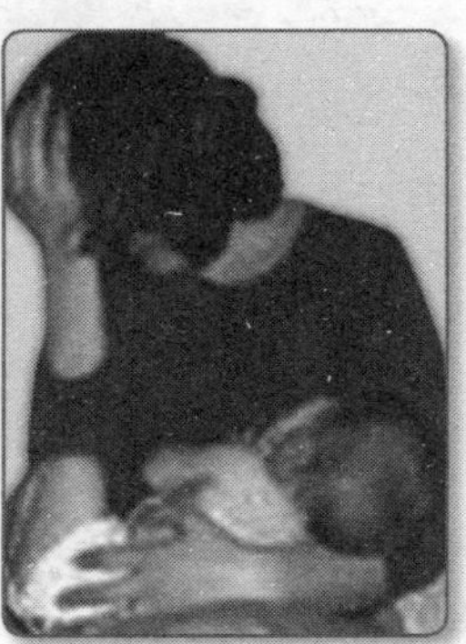

Fig. 9.8: It is painful

Then Advice the Mother

Advice her not to wash her breasts more than once a day, and to use soap, or rub hard with a towel. Breasts do not need to be washed before or after feeds. Normal washing as for the rest of the body is all that is necessary. Washing removes natural oils from the skin, and makes soreness more likely. Advice her not to use medicated lotions and ointments because these can irritate the skin, and there is no evidence that they are useful.

chapter 10

Not Accepting Breastfeed and Crying

Introduction

Many families start top milk because child refuses to feed. That leads to complete stopping of breastfeeding. If baby is "crying too much", mother and relatives think that the breast milk may be inadequate. She starts animal milk. We have to tell her about her baby's crying and refusal to feed (Fig. 10.1).

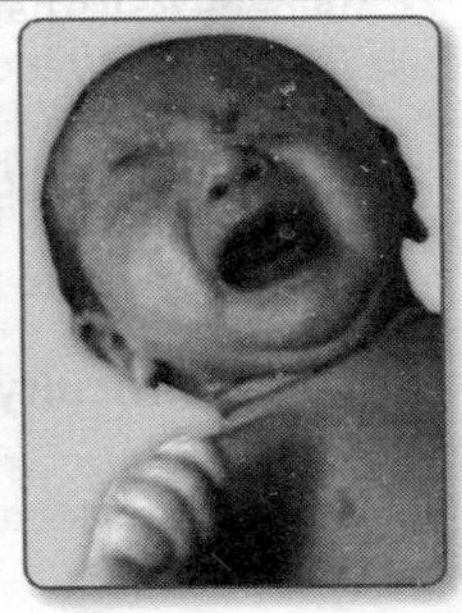

Fig. 10.1: Crying too much

Kinds of Refusal

There are different kinds of refusal:

- Sometimes a baby attaches to the breast, but then does not suckle or swallow, or suckles very weakly
- Sometimes a baby suckles for a minute and then comes off the breast chocking or crying. She/he may do this several times during a single feed
- Sometimes a baby takes one breast, but refuses the other
- A baby who cries a lot can upset the relationship between him/her and his/her mother and can cause tension among other family members.

You need to know how to decide why a baby is refusing to breastfeed, and how to help the mother and baby enjoy breastfeeding again.

Why A Baby May Refuse to Breastfeed?

Is the Baby Ill, in Pain or Sedated?

- *Illness:* The baby may attach to the breast, but suckles less than before.

- *Blocked nose:* Sore mouth [Candida infection (thrush)], an older baby teething. The baby suckles a few times, and then stops and cries.
- *Pain:* Pressure on a bruise from forceps or vacuum extraction. The baby cries and fights as his/her mother tries to breastfeed him.
- *Sedation:* A baby may be sleepy because of:
  - Drugs that his/her mother was given during delivery
  - Drugs that she is taking for psychiatric treatment
  - Drugs given to the baby.

Is there a Difficulty with the Breastfeeding Technique?

Sometimes breastfeeding has become unpleasant or frustrating for a baby.

Possible Causes

- Feeding from a bottle, or sucking on a pacifier (dummy)
- Not getting much milk, because of poor attachment or engorgement
- Pressure on the back of the baby's head, by his mother or a helper positioning him roughly, with poor technique. The pressure makes him/her want to "fight"
- His/her mother holding or shaking the breast, which interferes with attachment
- Restriction of breastfeeds; for example, breastfeeding only at certain times.

Has a Change Upset the Baby?

Babies have strong feeling, and if they are upset they may refuse to breastfeed. They may not cry but simply refuse to suckle. This is the most common when a baby is aged 3–12 months. She/he suddenly refuses several breastfeeds. This behavior is sometimes called a "nursing strike".

Possible Causes

- A new caretaker, or too many caretakers
- A change in the family routine, for example, moving house, visiting relatives

- Illness of his/her mother, or a breast infection
- His/her mother menstruating
- A change in his/her mother's smell, for example, different soap, or different food, different scent.

Is It "Apparent" and Not "Real" Refusal?

Sometimes a baby behaves in a way which makes his/her mother think that she/he is refusing to breastfeed. However, she/he is not really refusing. When a newborn baby "roots" for the breast, she/he moves his/her head from side to side as if she/he is saying "no". However, this is normal behavior. Between 4 and 8 months of age, babies are easily distracted, for example when they hear a noise. They may suddenly stop suckling. It is a sign that they are alert. After the age of 1 year, a baby may wean himself. This is usually gradual.

How to Help A Family with A Baby Who Refuses to Breastfeed or Cries A Lot?

Look for A Cause

Listen and Learn

- Help the mother to talk about how she feels. Empathize with her feelings

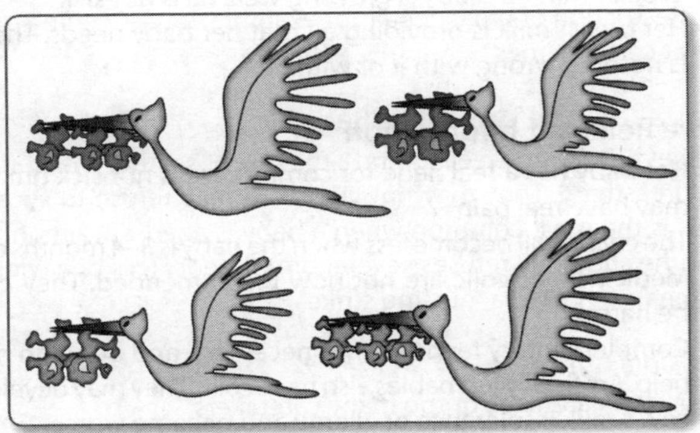

Fig. 10.2: Helping hand is important

- She may feel guilty and angry
- Other people may advise her to give the baby complements or pacifiers.

Take a History

- Baby's feeding and behavior
- Mother's diet, coffee, smoking and drugs
- Pressures from the family and other people
- Job work and general health of the mother.

Assess a Breastfeed

Check the baby's suckling position, skin of the breast, nipples and the length of a feed.

Examine the Baby

- Make sure he is not ill or in pain. Check his growth
- If the baby is ill or in pain, treat or refer as appropriate.

Build Confidence and Give Support

- Accept what the mother thinks about the cause of the problem
- Accept what she feels about the baby and his/her behavior.

Praise What the Mother and Baby are Doing Right

- Explain that her baby is growing well, he is not sick
- Her breast milk is providing all that her baby needs. There is nothing wrong with it or with her.

Give Relevant Information

- Her baby has a real need for comfort. He is not sick but he may have real pain
- The crying will become less when the baby is 3–4 months old
- Medicines for colic are not now recommended. They can be harmful
- Complementary feeds are not necessary, and often do not help. Artificially fed babies also have colic. They may develop cow's milk intolerance or allergy and become worse.

Make One or Two Suggestions

What you suggest depends on what you have learnt about the case of the crying. Common causes may be different in different countries.

If She Has an Oversupply of Breast Milk

Help her to improve her baby's attachment to the breast. Suggest that she lets him suckle from one breast only at each feed. Let him continue at the breast until he finishes by himself. Give the other breast at the next feed. Explain that if her baby stays on the first breast longer, he will get more fat-rich hindmilk.

Give Practical Help

- Explain that the best way to comfort a crying baby is to hold him close, with gentle movement and gentle pressure on his abdomen. Offer to show her some ways to hold and carry her baby
- Sometimes it is easier for someone not the mother to carry the baby so that he cannot smell the breast milk
- Show her how to bring up her baby's wind (called as burping). She should hold him upright, for example, in a sitting position or upright against her shoulder (Fig. 10.3)

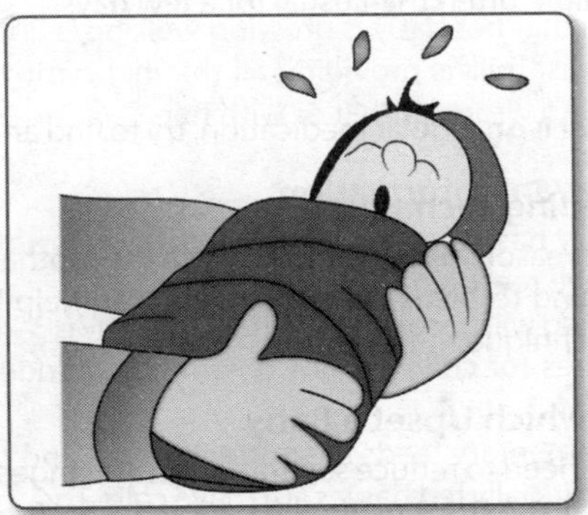

Fig. 10.3: Practical help

- Offer to discuss the situation with her family, to talk about the baby's needs and about her need for support
- It is important to try to help to reduce family tensions so that she does not start giving unnecessary complements.

Treat or Remove the Cause If Possible

Illness

- Treat infections with appropriate antimicrobials and other therapy
- Refer if necessary
- If a baby is unable to suckle, she/he may need special care in hospital
- Help his/her mother to express her breast milk to feed to him/her by cup.

Pain

- *For a bruise:* Help the mother to find a way to hold the baby without pressing on a painful place.
- *For thrush:* Treat with gentian violet or nystatin.
- *For teething:* Encourage her to be patient and to keep offering him her breast.
- *For a blocked nose:* Explain how she can clear it. Suggest short feeds, more often than usual for a few days.

Sedation

If the mother is on regular medication, try to find an alternative.

Breastfeeding Technique

Discuss the reason for the difficulty with the mother. When her baby is willing to breastfeed again; you can help her mother with her technique.

Changes which Upset a Baby

Discuss the need to reduce separation and changes if possible. Suggest that she stops using the new soap, perfume, or food.

If It Is a Distraction

Suggest that she try to feed him at a quiet place. The problem usually passes.

If It Is Self-weaning

Suggest that she makes sure that the child eats enough family food; give him plenty of extra-attention in other ways; continues to sleep with him because night feeds may continue (Fig. 10.4). This is valuable at least up to the age of 2 years.

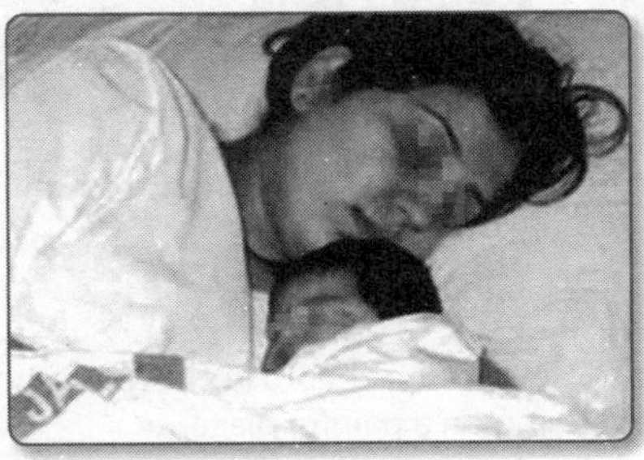

Fig. 10.4: Sedated mother gets problems

Expressing Breast Milk

chapter 11

Introduction

Expressing breast milk is useful in many situations. The skill of expressing breast milk is important as it enables a mother to initiate or continue breastfeeding (Fig. 11.1).

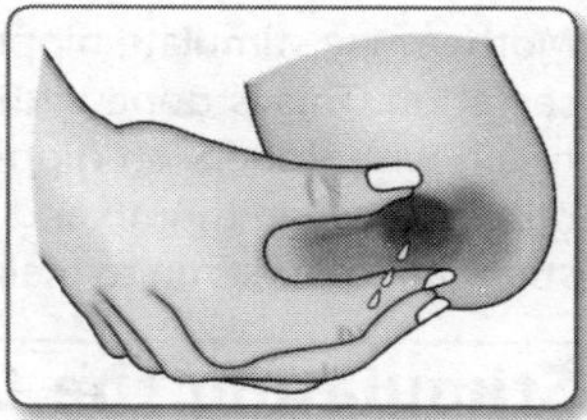

Fig. 11.1: Milk expression from breast

Expressing Breast Milk

Expressing milk is useful to:

- Relieve engorgement
- Relieve blocked duct or milk stasis
- Feed a baby while she/he learns to suckle from an inverted nipple
- Feed a baby who has difficulty in coordinating suckling
- Feed a baby who "refuses", while he learns to enjoy breastfeeding
- Feed a low birth weight baby who cannot breastfeed
- Feed a sick baby, who cannot suckle enough
- Keep up the supply of breast milk when a mother or baby is ill
- Leave breast milk for a baby when his mother goes out or to work
- Prevent leaking when a mother is away from her baby
- Help a baby to attach to a full breast
- Express breast milk directly into a baby's mouth
- Prevent the nipple and areola from becoming dry and sore.

The most useful way for a mother to express milk is by hand. It needs no appliance, so she can do it anywhere and at any time. With a good technique, it can be very efficient. It is easy to hand express when the breasts are soft.

Before one learns expression of breast milk it is important to know what are the other ways to stimulate hormones necessary for milk secretion (prolactin) and milk flow (oxytocin).

Stimulating Prolactin (Milk Secretion) Reflex

Mother may stimulate nipple and areola to help in prolactin secretion. This is done with a gentle stroke on breast, light touch with fingers on nipple, areola and by gently rubbing nipple between thumb and index finger. It is wise to keep on stimulating prolactin to maintain milk secretion (Fig. 11.2).

Stimulating the Oxytocin (Milk Flow) Reflex

The oxytocin reflex works well when a baby suckles. It may not work well, when she expresses milk.

How to Stimulate the Oxytocin Reflex?

Help the mother psychologically:

- Build here confidence
- Try to reduce any sources of pain or anxiety
- Help her to have good thoughts and feeling about the baby.

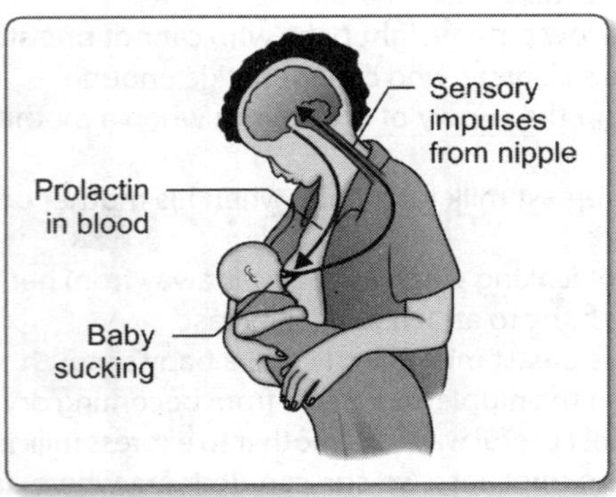

Fig. 11.2: Prolactin reflex

Help the mother practically. Help or advice her to:

- *Sit quietly and privately or with a supportive friend:* Some mothers can express easily in a group.
- *Hold her baby with skin to skin contact:* She can hold her baby on her lap while she expresses. If this is not possible, she can look at the baby. If this is not possible, sometimes even looking at a photograph of her baby helps.
- *Warm her breasts:* For example, she can apply a warm compress or warm water, or have a warm shower.
- *Stimulate her nipples:* She can gently pull or roll her nipples with her fingers.
- *Massage or stroke the breasts lightly:* Some women find that it helps if they stroke the nipple and areola gently with fingertips or with a comb. Some women find that it helps to gently roll their closed fist over the breast toward the thumbs pointing forward.
- *Ask a helper to rub her back:* The mother sits down, leans forward, folds her arms on a table in front of her, and rests her head on arms. Her breasts hang loose, unclothed. The helper rubs down both sides of the mother's spine. She uses her closed fist with her small circular movements with her thumbs. She works down both sides of the spine at the same time, form the neck to the shoulder blades, for 2 or 3 minutes (Figs 11.3A and B).

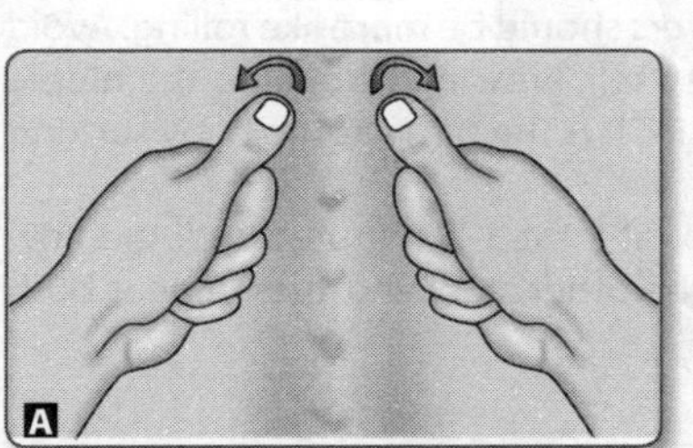

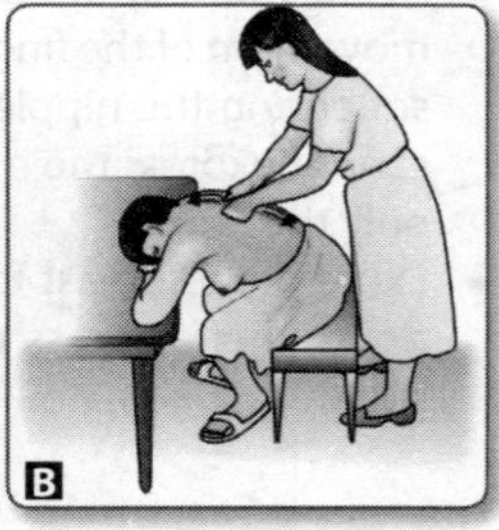

Figs 11.3A and B: (A and B) A helper rubbing a mother's back to stimulate the oxytocin reflex

How to Express Breast Milk by Hand?

Teach a mother to do this herself. Do not express her milk for her. Touch her only to show her what to do. Be gentle. Teach her to:

- Wash her hands thoroughly
- Sit or stand comfortably
- Hold the container near her breast
- Put her thumb on her breast above the nipple and areola, and her first finger on the breast below the nipple and areola, opposite the thumb. She supports the breast with her other fingers
- Press her thumb and first finger slightly inward toward the chest wall. She should avoid pressing too far, because that can block the milk ducts
- Press her breast behind the nipple and areola between her finger and thumb. She must press on the lactiferous sinuses beneath the areola. Sometimes in a lactating breast, it is possible to feel the sinuses. They are like peanuts. If she can feel them, she can press on them
- Press and release, again press and release. This should not hurt. If it hurts, the technique is wrong. At first no milk may come, but after pressing a few times milk starts to drip out. It may flow in streams if the oxytocin reflex is active
- Press the areola in the same way from the sides, to make sure that milk is expressed from all segments of the breast
- Avoid rubbing or sliding her fingers along the skin. The movement of the fingers should be more like rolling. Avoid squeezing the nipple itself. Pressing or pulling the nipple cannot express the milk. It is the same as the baby sucking only the nipple
- Express one breast for at least 3–5 minutes until the flow slows; then express the other side; and then repeat both sides.

Explain that to express breast milk adequately takes 20–30 minutes, especially in the first few days when only a little milk may be produced. It is important not to try to express in a shorter time.

How Often A Mother Should Express Milk?

To Establish Lactation, to Feed a Low Birth Weight (LBW) or Sick Newborn

She should start to express milk on the first day, within 6 hours of delivery if possible. She may only express a few drops of colostrum at first, but it helps breast milk production to begin, in the same way, that baby suckling soon after delivery helps breast milk production to begin.

To Keep Up Her Milk Supply to Feed a Sick Baby

She should express as much as she can as often as her baby would feed, at least every 3 hours.

To Relieve Symptoms, Such As Engorgement or Leaking at Work

Express only as much as is necessary.

To Leave Milk for a Baby while She is Out at Work

Express as much as possible before she goes to work, and to leave milk for the baby. It is also very important to express while at work to help keep up the supply.

Breast Pump

If hand expression is difficult, a mother can use a hand breast pump.

Rubber Bulb Pump

Rubber bulb pumps are not very efficient, especially when the breasts are soft. They are not suitable for collecting milk to feed a baby. They are difficult to clean properly. Milk may collect in the rubber bulb and it is difficult to clean out. The milk, which collects, is often contaminated.

Syringe Pump

Syringe pumps are more efficient than rubber bulb pumps. They are easier to clean and sterilize.

How to Use a Syringe Pump

- Put the plunger inside the outer cylinder
- Make sure that the rubber seal is in good flexible condition
- Put the funnel over the nipple, make sure that it touches the skin all round
- To make an airtight seal, pull the outer cylinder down
- The nipple is sucked into the funnel
- Release the outer cylinder, and pull down again
- After a minute or two, milk starts to flow and collects in outer cylinder. When milk stops flowing, break the seal, pour out the milk and then repeat the procedure.

chapter 12

Inadequate Milk

Introduction

Almost all mothers can produce enough breast milk for one or even two babies. Usually even when a mother thinks that she does not have enough breast milk, her baby is in a fact getting all that she/he needs.

Sometimes, a baby does not get enough breast milk. But it is usually because she/he is not suckling enough or not sucking effectively. It is rarely because his/her mother cannot produce enough milk.

So it is important to think not about how much milk a mother can produce, but about how much milk a baby is getting.

Signs that A Baby may Not Be Getting Enough Breast Milk

Reliable

- Poor weight gain (<500 grams a month) (< birth weight after 2 weeks)
- Passing small amount of concentrated urine (<6 times a day).

Possible

- Baby not satisfied after breastfeeds
- Baby cries often
- Very frequent breastfeeds
- Very long breastfeeds
- Baby refuses to breastfeed
- Baby has hard, dry or green stools

- No milk comes when mother tries to express
- Breasts did not enlarge (during pregnancy)
- Milk did not "come in" (after delivery).

How to Find out If A Baby is Getting Enough Breast Milk or Not

Check the Baby's Weight Gain

This is the most reliable sign. For the first 6 months of life, a baby should gain at least 500 g in weight each month or 125 g each week (one kilogram per month is not necessary and not usual). If a baby gains less than 500 g in a month, she/he is not gaining enough weight. Look at the baby's growth chart if available, or at any other record of previous weights. If no weight record is available, weigh the baby. If the baby is gaining enough weight, she/he is getting enough milk. However, if no weight record is available, you cannot get an immediate answer.

Check the Baby's Urine Output

This is a useful quick check. An exclusively breastfed baby who is getting enough milk usually passes dilute urine at least 6–8 times in 24 hours. A baby who is not getting enough breast milk passes urine less than 6 times a day (often less than 4 times a day) (Fig. 12.1).

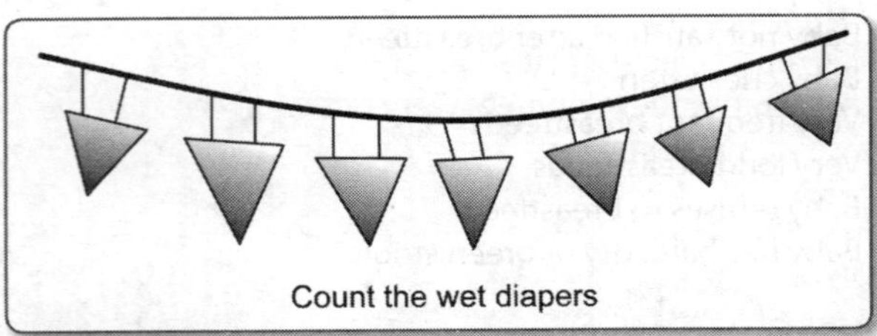

Fig. 12.1: Wet diappers

Reasons for Baby Not Getting Enough Milk

Breastfeeding Factors

- Delayed start, poor support
- Poor attachment
- Feeding at fixed times
- Infrequent feeds
- No night feeds
- Short feeds
- Bottles, pacifiers
- Other foods
- Other fluids (water, teas).

These are common.

Mother: Psychological Factor

- Lack of confidence
- Worry, stress
- Dislike of breastfeeding
- Rejection of baby
- Tiredness.

Mother: Physical Condition

- Contraception pill, diuretics
- Pregnancy
- Severe malnutrition
- Alcohol
- Smoking
- Retained piece of placenta (rare)
- Poor breast development (very rare).

These are not common.

Baby's Condition

- Low birth weight
- Nose block illness
- Cleft lip or palate
- Other abnormalities
- Oral thrush

Factors that Do Not Affect the Breast Milk Supply

- Age of the mother
- Sexual intercourse
- Menstruation
- Age of baby
- Cesarean section.

If a baby passes lot of urine, it usually means that she/he is getting plenty of breast milk.

How to Increase Breast Milk and Relactation?

chapter 13

Introduction

If a mother's breast milk supply is reduced, she needs to increase it. If a mother has stopped breastfeeding, she may want to start again. This is called relactation (Fig. 13.1).

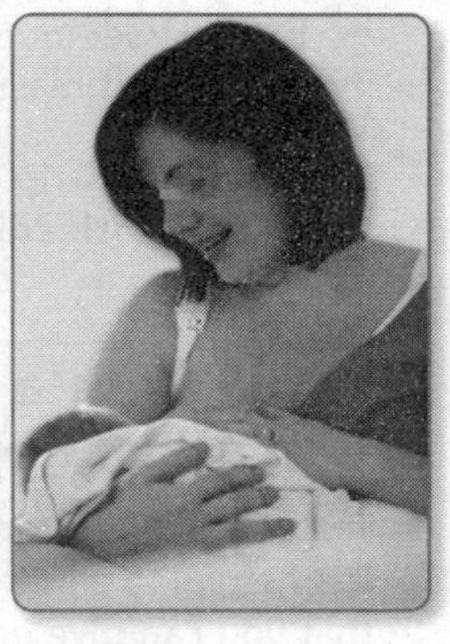

Fig. 13.1: Relactation

The situations in which mothers may want to relactate include when:

- A baby has been sick and has not suckled for a time
- A baby has been artificially fed, but now the mother wants to try breastfeeding
- The mother has been sick and stopped feeding her baby
- A woman adopts a baby.

The same principles and methods apply for increasing a reduced supply, and for relactation. However, relactation is more difficult and takes longer. The mother must be well motivated and she needs a lot of support to succeed. Sometimes it is also necessary to use the methods described in Management of Refusal to Breastfeed.

How to Help a Mother to Increase Her Milk?

She must let her baby suckle often to stimulate her breast. If her baby does not suckle often, her breast milk will not increase whatever else she does. Eating more does not by itself increase a women's milk supply. However, if she is undernourished, she needs to eat more to build up her strength and energy. If she is not undernourished, food and warm nourishing drinks may help her to feel confident and relaxed. Many mothers notice that they are more thirsty than usual when they are breastfeeding, especially near the time of a feed. They should drink to satisfy their thirst. However, taking more fluid than they feel for their need does not increase their breast milk supply. In most communities, experienced women know of some form of lactogogue. Lactogogues are special foods, drinks or herbs which people believe to increase the breast milk supply. They do not work like drugs, but may help a woman to feel confident and relaxed.

- **The Drop and Drip Technique (Fig. 13.2)**
- **Using a Breastfeeding Supplementer (13.3)**

How to Help a Woman to Increase Her Breast Milk Supply?

- Try to help mother and baby at home if possible. Sometimes it is helpful to admit them to hospital for a week or two so that you can give enough help—especially if the mother may feel pressure to use a bottle again at home
- Discuss with the mother the reason for her poor milk supply. Explain what she needs to do to increase her supply. Explain that it takes patience and perseverance

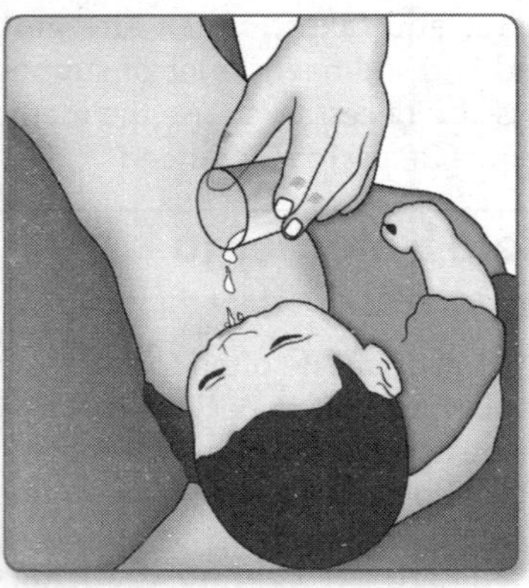

Fig. 13.2: The drop and drip technique

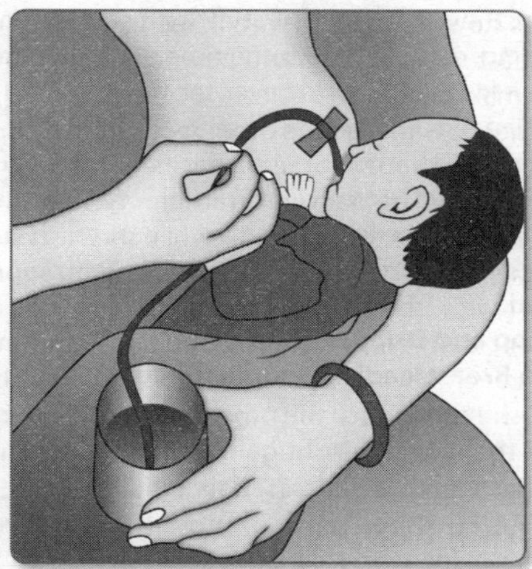

Fig. 13.3: Using a breastfeeding supplementer

- Use all the ways you have learnt to build her confidence. Help her to feel that she can produce breast milk again or increase her supply. Try to see her and talk to her often at least twice a day. Make sure that she has enough to eat and drink
- If you know of a locally valued lactogogue, encourage her to take that
- Encourage her to rest more, and to try to relax when she breastfeeds
- Explain that she should keep her baby near her; give him plenty of skin to skin contact
- Explain that the most important thing is to let baby suckle more at least 10 times in 24 hours, more if she/he is willing. She/he can offer her breast every 2 hours. She/he should let him/her suckle whenever she/he seems interested. She/he should let him/her suckle longer than before at each breast. She/he should keep him/her with her and breastfeed at night. Sometimes it is easiest to get a baby to suckle when she/he is sleepy
- Make sure that her baby attaches well to the breast

- Discuss how to give other milk feeds, while she waits for her breast milk to come, and how to reduce the other milk as her milk increases
- Show her how to give the other feeds from a cup, not from a bottle. She should not use a pacifier
- If her baby refuses to suckle on an "empty" breast, help her to find a way to give the baby milk while she/he is suckling. For example, with a dropper or a breastfeeding supplementer
- To start with, she should give the full amount of artificial feed for a baby of his weight or the same amount that she/he has been having before. As soon as a little breast milk come, she can reduce the other milk by 30–60 ml each day
- Check the baby's weight gain and urine output, to make sure that she/he is getting enough milk.
  - If she/he is not getting enough, do not reduce the artificial feed for a few days
  - If necessary, increase the amount of artificial milk for a day or two.

Some women can decrease the amount by more than 30–60 ml each day.

If as a counselor, you are not motivated and committed to relactation, you will not be able to motivate the mother. "Lactation failure", in fact, is not failure of the mother; it is the failure of her "adviser".

How to Help a Mother to use a Breastfeeding Supplementer?

Show the mother how to:

- Use a fine nasogastric tube or other fine plastic tubing and a cup to hold the milk. If there is no very fine tube, use the best available
- Cut a small hole in the side of the tube, near the end of the part that goes into the baby's mouth (this is in addition to the hole at the end)
- Prepare a cup of milk (expressed breast milk or artificial milk) containing the amount of milk that her baby needs for one feed

- Put one end of the tube along her nipple so that her baby suckles the breast and the tube at the same time. Tape the tube in place on her breast
- Put the other end of the tube into the cup of milk
- Tie a knot in the tube if it is wide, or put a paper clip on it, or pinch it. This controls the flow of milk so that her baby does not finish the feed too fast
- Control the flow of milk so that her baby suckles for about 30 minutes at each feed if possible (raising the cup makes the milk flow faster, lowering the cup makes the milk flow more slowly)
- Let her baby suckle at many times that she/he is willing—not just when she is using the supplementer
- Clean and sterilize the tube of the supplementer and the cup or bottle, each time she uses them.

[illegible] to increase breast milk production.

- Put one end of the tube along the breast so that the baby suckles the breast and the tube at the same time. Tape the tube in place on the breast.
- Put the other end of the tube into the cup of milk.
- [illegible] the tube [illegible] the baby [illegible] not finish the feed too fast.
- Control the flow of milk so that the baby suckles for about 30 minutes [illegible] the milk flow [illegible] lowering the cup makes the milk flow [illegible] slowly)
- Let the baby suckle [illegible] the supplementer.
- Clean and sterilize the tube of the supplementer and the cup [illegible] time you use them.

chapter 14

Preparation of Top Feeds

Introduction

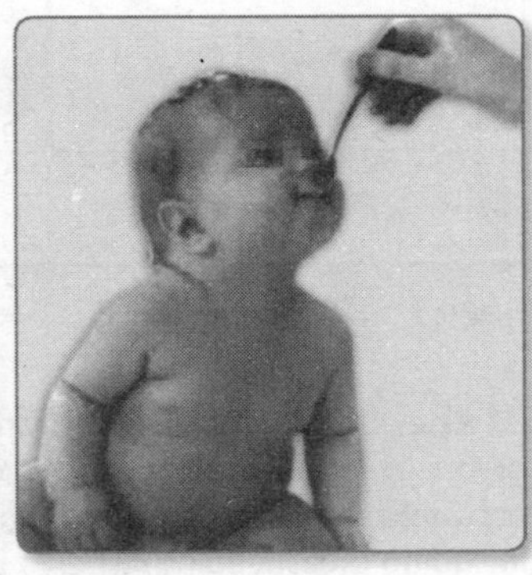

Fig. 14.1: Top feeding

Many families start top feeds: (1) on their own, (2) on their doctor's advice or (3) some HIV positive mothers choose not to give breast milk. Mothers and other caregivers need to know how to prepare replacement feeds for their infants. Feeds must be prepared in safest possible way, to reduce the risk of illness.

In this chapter, we discuss how: to make measures for liquids and powders to make measures using utensils that a mother brings from home; to prepare feeds of recipes given, using home measures.

How the mother makes feeds, whether from commercial formula (try to avoid) or home prepared, it is very important that the milk and water are mixed in the correct amounts, and also sugar and micronutrients added if needed. Wrongly prepared feeds make a baby ill, or she/he may be underfed.

The amount of milk that a baby takes at each feed varies. But the caregiver must decide how much to put in a cup to offer the baby. A baby needs an average of 150 ml/kg per day. This is divided into 6, 7 or 8 feeds (Fig. 14.1).

Approximate Amount of Formula Needed Per Day

The approximate amount of formula needed per day has been shown in Table 14.1.

Age (months)	*Weight (kg)*	*Approximate amount of formula per 24 hours (ml)*	*Approximate number of feeds (ml)*
1st	3	450	8 x 60
2nd	4	600	7 x 90
3rd	5	750	6 x 120
4th	5.5	750	6 x 120
5th	69	900	6 x 150
6th	6.5	900	6 x 150

Table 14.1: The approximate amount of formula needed per day

A newborn infant is fed small amounts frequently. The amount gradually increases as the infant grows. Amount of milk that a baby takes at each feed varies, whatever the method of feeding, including breastfeeding. When a baby is feeding by cup, offer a little extra, but let the baby decide when to stop. If a baby takes a very small feed, offer extra at the next feed, or give the next feed earlier, especially if the baby shows signs of hunger.

Approximate Amount of Milk Needed by Month

The approximate amount of milk needed by month has been shown in Table 14.2.

- Commercial formulas should be avoided
- Exclusive breastfeeding till 6 months.

How to Measure Sugar and Milk Powder?

You can measure sugar by spoon or by weight. Most mothers find it easier to use a spoon than to measure small weights like 8 g (Fig. 14.2). However, spoons differ in size.

Ask a mother to bring a spoon from home so that you can show her how to measure with that spoon. She should try to

Age (months)	*Milk feeds (ml/ day)*	*Cow's milk, water and sugar needed to make home prepared formula per day*	*Commercial formula needed per month (g tins)*
1st	450	300 ml milk + 150 ml water + 30 g sugar	4 x 500
2nd	600	400 ml milk + 200 ml water + 40 g sugar	6 x 500
3rd	750	500 ml milk + 250 ml water + 45 g sugar	7 x 500
4th	750	575 ml milk + 250 ml water + 45 g sugar	7 x 500
5th	900	600 ml milk + 300 ml water + 56 g sugar	8 x 500
6th	975	675 ml milk + 300 ml water + 56 g sugar	40 x 500 (20 kg)

Table 14.2: The approximate amount of milk needed by month

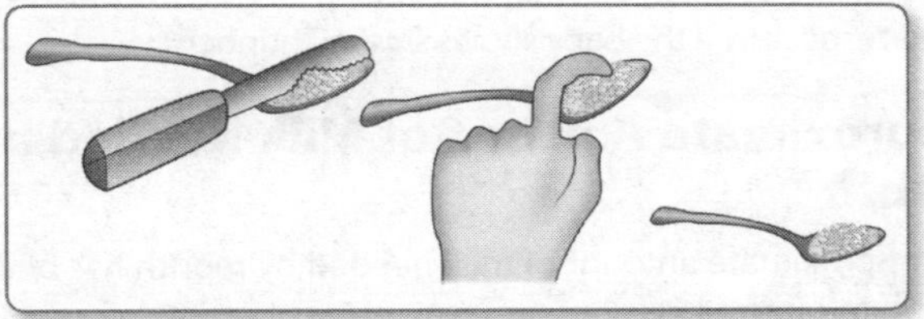

Fig. 14.2: Measuring sugar by spoon

keep this same spoon especially for making up feeds for her baby.

You need to know how full to make each size of spoon to measure 8 g. There are three ways to fill a spoon: (1) level it with the back of a knife or handle of another spoon (2) "round" the spoon (with curved finger) and (3) heap the spoon. For smaller amounts, you can make a level spoonful and then take away half the sugar.

How to use Commercial Infant Formula?

Strict training of the mother is essential before recommending powder milk formula. Usually commercial infant formula comes with special measures (called a scoop) in the tin of powder. This should be used only for that brand of infant formula. Different brands may have different size measures. Scoops always have to be leveled. Use the quantities printed on the label. Generally 1 ounce water (30 ml) needs 1 scoop of commercial milk powder. Likewise 120 ml water need 4 level scoops of commercial milk powder.

Breastfeeding Low Birth Weight and Sick Babies

chapter 15

Introduction

The term low birth weight (LBW) means a birth weight of less than 2,500 grams (Fig. 15.1). A LBW may be premature or small for gestational age or both. In many countries, 15–20% of all babies are LBW. In India, 30% of all babies are LBW. Preterm babies need more of some nutrients, e.g. proteins, sodium, calcium and some of amino acids like taurine, cystine and essential fatty acids and carnitine than mature breast milk can provide. Two-thirds of the low birth babies in developing countries are small for date.

Low birth weight babies need breast milk even more than larger babies. The best milk for a LBW baby is his/her own mother's milk. Preterm milk is specially adapted to the needs of a preterm baby. It contains extra protein and extra anti-infective factors.

How to Help Breastfeeding if a Baby is Low Birth Weight?

For the first few days, a baby may not be able to take any oral feeds. She/he may need to be fed intravenously. Oral feeds should begin as soon as the baby tolerates them.

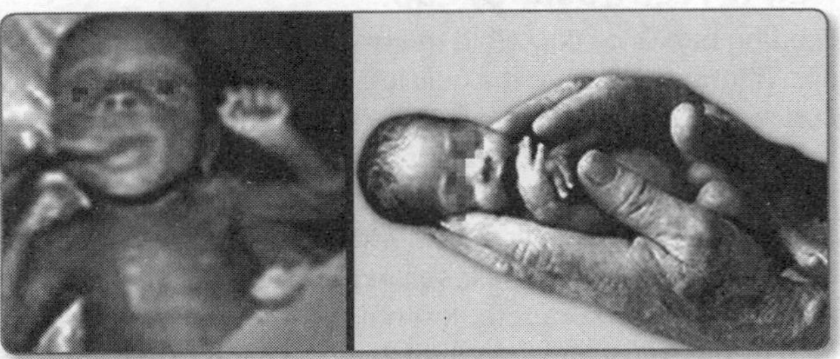

Fig. 15.1: Low birth weight baby

Babies who are less than about 32 weeks of gestational age usually need to be fed by nasogastric tube. Give expressed breast milk (EBM) by tube.

Babies between about 32 and 34 weeks of gestational age can take feeds from a small cup, or from a spoon. You can start trying to give cup feeds once or twice a day while a baby is still having most of his/her feeds by tube. If she/he takes cup feeds well, you can reduce the tube feeds.

Babies of about 34 weeks of gestational age or more are able to start suckling on the breast. Let the mother put her/his baby to her breast as soon as she/he is well enough. She/he may only root for the nipple and lick it at first, or she/he may suckle a little. Continue giving EBM by cup or tube, to make sure that the baby gets all that she/he needs.

When a LBW baby starts to suckle effectively, she/he may pause quite often during feeds, to breathe. It is important to leave him/her on the breast so that she/he can suckle again when she/he is ready. Offer a cup feed after the breastfeed. Or offer alternative breast and cup feeds. Make sure that the baby suckles in a good position. Good attachment may make effective suckling possible at an earlier stage.

Babies from about 34 to 36 weeks of gestational age or more can usually take all that they need directly from the breast. Supplements from a cup are no longer necessary. Continue to follow babies up and weigh them regularly to make sure that they are getting all the breast milk that they need.

How to Feed a Baby by Cup?

Feeding babies by cup: Hold the small cup of milk to the baby's lips. Tilt the cup so that the milk just reaches the baby's lips. The cup rests lightly on the baby's lower lip, and the edges of the cup touch the outer part of the baby's upper lip. The baby becomes alert, and opens his/her mouth and eyes. A LBW baby starts to take the milk into his/her mouth with his/her tongue. A full term or older baby sucks the milk, spilling some of it. Do not pour the milk into the baby's mouth. Just hold the cup to his/her lips and let him/her take it himself. When the baby has had enough, she/he closes his/her mouth and will not take any more. If she/he has

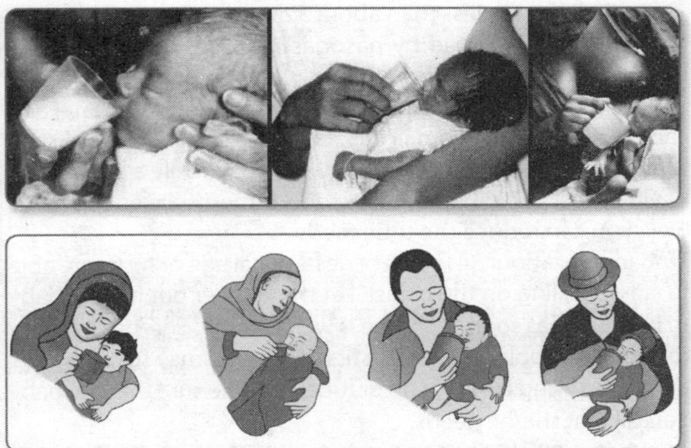

Fig. 15.2: Methods to feed sick babies

not taken the calculated amount, she/he may take more next time or you may need to feed him/her more often. Measure his/her intake over 24 hours—not just at each feed.

How to Help Breastfeeding if a Baby is Sick ?

Babies who are sick recover more quickly if they continue to take breast milk during the illness (Figs 15.2 and 15.3).

If a Baby is in the Hospital

Admit his/her mother too so that she can stay with him/her and breastfeed him/her.

If a Baby Can Suckle Well

Encourage his/her mother to breastfeed more often. She can increase the number of feeds up to 12 times a day or more when she/he is sick. Sometimes a baby loses his/her appetite for other foods, but continues to want to breastfeed. This is quite common with children who have diarrhea. Sometimes a baby likes to breastfeed more when she/he is ill than before, and this can increase the supply of breast milk

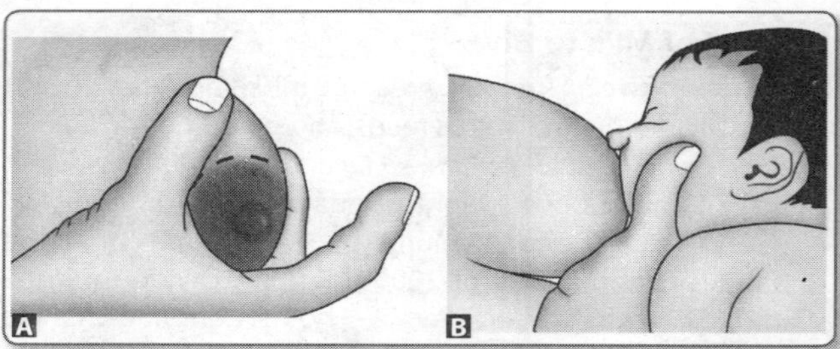

Figs 15.3A and B: The dancer hand position to help a baby with muscular weakness to attach to the breast. (A) The mother supports her breast with the plam of her hand and the three outer fingers; (B) Her finger and thumb are free to support the baby's chin and cheeks

If a Baby Suckles, But Less than before at Each Feed

Suggest that his/her mother may give in more frequent feeds, even if they are shorter (small frequent feeds). Help his/her mother to express her milk, and give it by cup. Let the baby continue to suckle when she/he is willing. Even babies on intravenous fluids may be able to suckle, or to have EBM.

If a Baby is Unable to Take Expressed Milk from a Cup

It may be necessary to give the EBM through a nasogastric tube for a few feeds.

Amount of Milk for Babies Who cannot Breastfeed

What Milk to Give

- *Choice 1*: Expressed breast milk (if possible from the baby's mother)
- *Choice 2*: Formula made up according to the instructions
- *Choice 3*: Animal milk (dilute cow's milk with 1 cup of water to 2 cups milk, and add 1 level teaspoon of sugar to each cup of feed. This is called as humanization of cow's milk.)

Amount of Milk to Give

- *Babies who weigh 2.5 kg or more*: 150 ml/kg body weight per day. Divide the total into 8 feeds, and give 3 hourly.
- *Babies who weigh less than 2.5 kg or less (low birth weight)*: 60–200 ml/kg body weight per day. Start with 60 ml/kg/day. Increase the total volume by 20 ml/kg/day, until the baby is taking a total of 200 ml/kg/day. Divide the total into 8–12 feeds, to feed every 2–3 hours. Continue until the baby weighs 1,800 grams or more, and is fully breastfeeding. Check the baby's 24-hours intake. The size of individual feeds may vary.

chapter 16

Kangaroo Mother Care

Introduction

Kangaroo mother care (KMC) is a way to care for the preterm infants. The infant is carried in skin to skin contact with the mother. It is a powerful and an easy to use method to promote the health and well-being of infants born preterm as well as full term (Figs 16.1A and B).

The key features are:

- Early continuous and prolonged skin to skin contact between the mother and the baby (Figs 16.2A and B)
- Exclusive breastfeeding
- It is initiated in the hospital and can be continued at home
- Small babies can be discharged early.

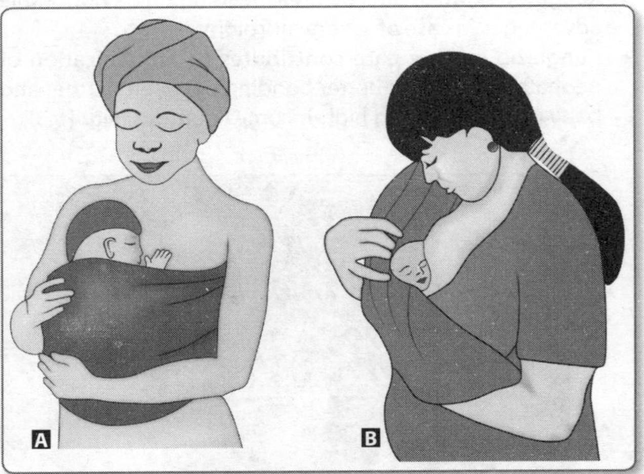

Figs 16.1A and B: Kangaroo mother care

Increased
adjustability
Smaller & lighter
shoulder pad
No hard edges
on the arm
Lighter &
softer rail
padding
A
B

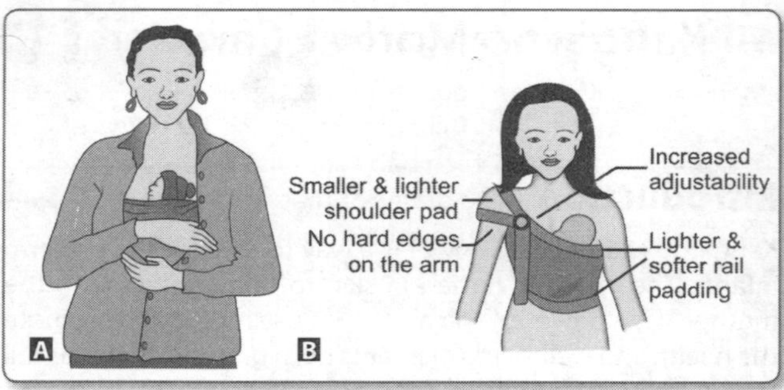

Figs 16.2A and B: (A) Baby in kangaroo mother care position; (B) new improved Sling EZee baby sling

Research and experience show that:

- Kangaroo mother care is at least equivalent to conventional incubator care, in terms of safety and thermal protection, as measured by mortality
- Kangaroo mother care, by breastfeeding offers noticeable advantages in case of severe morbidity
- Kangaroo mother care contributes to humanization of neonatal care and to better bonding between mother and baby in both low- and high-income countries (Fig. 16.3).

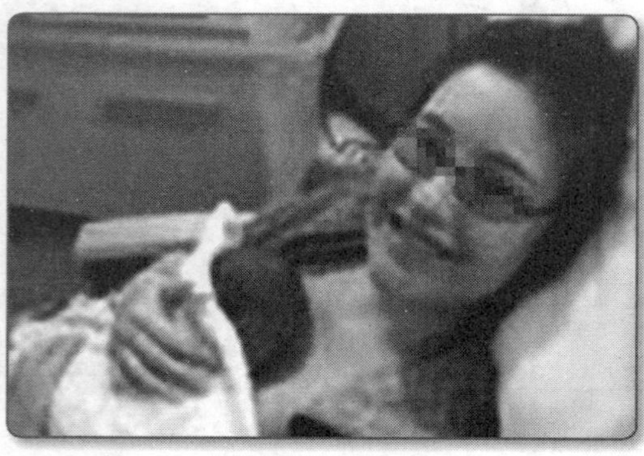

Fig. 16.3: Position of baby for kangaroo mother care

When to Start Kangaroo Mother Care?

When exactly KMC can begin for those small babies must be judged individually and full account should be taken of the condition and status of each baby and his/her mother.

Babies weighing 1,800 grams or more at birth (gestational age 30–34 weeks or more) may have some prematurity-related problems such as *respiratory distress syndrome* (RDS). This may raise serious concerns for a minority of those infants, who will require care in special units in most cases; however, KMC can start soon after birth.

In babies with birth weight between 1,200 and 1,799 grams, prematurity-related problems such as RDS and other complications are frequent. Therefore, they require some kind of special treatment initially. In such case, the delivery should take place in well-equipped facility, which could provide the care required. Should the delivery take place elsewhere, the baby should be transferred after birth, preferably with the mother. The best way of transporting small babies is keeping them in continuous skin to skin contact with the mother. It might take a week or more before KMC can be initiated.

Babies weighing less than 1,200 grams (gestational age below 30 weeks) incur frequent and severe problems due to preterm birth: mortality is very high and only a small percentage survives prematurity-related problems. These babies benefit most from transfer before birth to an institution with neonatal intensive care facilities.

Kangaroo Position

Place the baby between the mother's breasts in upright position, chest to chest (Fig. 16.4). Secure him/her with the binder. The head, turned to one side, is in a slightly extended position. The top of the binder is just under baby's ear. This slightly extended head position keeps the ear way open and allows eye to eye contact between the mother and the baby. Avoid both forward flexion and hyperextension of the head. The hips should be flexed and extended in a "frog" position; the arms should also be flexed.

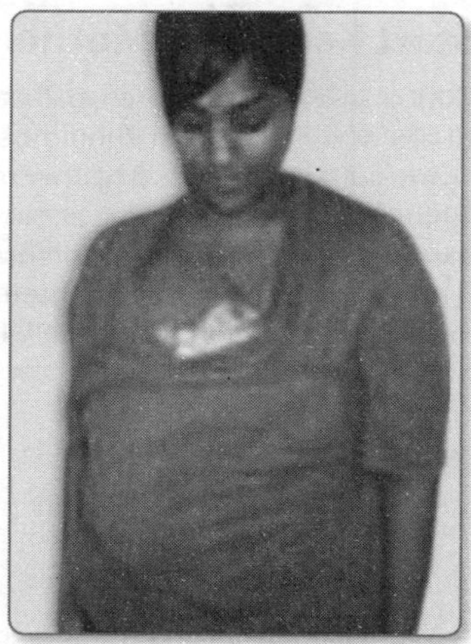

Fig. 16.4: Kangaroo position

Tie the cloth should be wrapped firmly enough so that when the mother stands up, the baby does not slide out. Make sure that the tight part of the cloth is over the baby's chest. Baby's abdomen should not be constricted and should be somewhere at the level of the mother epigastrium. This way baby has enough room for abdominal breathing. Mother's breathing stimulates the baby.

Duration

When the mother and baby are comfortable, skin to skin contact continues for as long as possible. Kangaroo position needs to be used until the baby reaches term. Around that time the baby also outgrows the need for KMC. Weaning from KMC can be started when baby is uncomfortable, pulls his/her limbs out, cries and fusses every time the mother tries to put her baby skin to skin. KMC at home is particularly important in cold climates or during the cold seasons and could go on for longer.

Length

Skin to skin contact should start gradually, with a smooth transition from conventional care to continuous KMC. Sessions that last less than 60 minutes should, however, be avoided because frequent changes are too stressful for baby. The length of skin to skin contacts gradually increases to become as continuous as possible, day and night, interrupted only for changing diapers, especially where no other means of thermal control are available.

Staffing

Kangaroo mother care does not require any more staff than conventional care. Existing staff (doctors and nurses) should have basic training in breastfeeding and adequate training in all aspects of KMC as described below:

- When and how to initiate the KMC method
- How to position baby between and during feeds
- Feeding LBW and preterm infants
- Breastfeeding
- Involving the mother in all aspects of her baby's care including monitoring vital signs and recognizing danger signs
- Taking timely and appropriate action when a problem is detected or the mother is concerned
- Deciding on discharge.

Monitoring Baby's Condition

Temperature

A well baby, in continuous skin to skin contact, can easily retain normal body temperature when in kangaroo position, if the ambient temperature is not lower than the recommended range. Hypothermia is rare in KMC infants, but it can occur. Measuring baby's body temperature is still needed, but less frequently than when the baby is not in the kangaroo position.

Observing Breathing and Well-Being

The normal respiratory rate of an LBW and preterm infant ranges between 30 and 60 breaths per minute. Breathing alternates with intervals of no breathing (apnea). However, if the interval becomes too long (20 seconds or more) and the baby's lips and face turn blue (cyanosis), his pulse is abnormally low (bradycardia) and he does not resume breathing spontaneously, act quickly: there is a risk of brain damage. The smaller or more premature the baby is, the longer and more frequent the spells of apnea.

What to Do in Case of Apnea

- Teach her to stimulate the baby by lightly rubbing the back or head, and by rocking movements until the baby starts breathing again. If the baby is still not breathing, she calls staff
- Always react immediately to a mother's call for help
- In case of prolonged apnea, when the breathing cannot be restarted through stimulation, resuscitate according to the hospital resuscitation guidelines
- If apneic spells become more frequent, examine the baby. This may be an early sign of infection, treat accordingly.

Danger Signs

- Difficulty in breathing, chest in-drawing, grunting
- Breathing very fast or very slow
- Frequent and long spells of apnea
- Baby feels cold. Body temperature is below normal despite rewarming
- Difficulty in feeding: the baby does not wake up for feeds anymore, stops feeding or vomits
- Convulsions
- Diarrhea
- Yellow skin.

Benefits of Kangaroo Mother Care

- *Breastfeed*: It appears that KMC and skin to skin contact are beneficial for breastfeeding in settings where it is less commonly used for the preterm or LBW infants. Earlier the KMC is begun and earlier skin to skin contact is initiated, the greater the effect on breastfeeding will be.
- *Growth*: KMC infant showed a slightly larger daily weight gain.
- *Thermal control and metabolism*: Prolonged skin to skin contact between the mother and her preterm or LBW infant as in KMC provides effective thermal control and reduced risk of hypothermia.
- *Other effects*: Heart rate, respiratory rate, oxygenation, oxygen consumption, blood glucose, sleep patterns and behavior observed in preterm or LBW infants held skin to skin tend to be similar to or better than those observed in infants separated from their mothers. Stress levels in babies also decrease as shown by decreased salivary cortisol levels.

chapter 17

HIV and Infant Feeding

Introduction

Risk of HIV Transmission Through Breastfeeding

The following diagram (Fig. 17.1) helps to explain the risks of mother-to-child transmission (MTCT). It shows 100 breastfeeding women from a population where HIV is highly prevalent.

The 2006 guidelines for HIV and infant feeding suggested that health workers should individually counsel all HIV positive mothers to help them each determine, the most appropriate infant feeding strategy, in their circumstances. However, the 2009 recommendations state that national health authorities should promote a single infant feeding practice as the standard of care. Based on various conditions like (i) international recommendations, (ii) socioeconomics (iii) cultural contexts of the country's population, (iv) the availability and quality of health services, (v) the local epidemiology including HIV prevalence among pregnant women and (vi) main cause of infant mortality and undernutrition.

This strategy will give infants the greatest chance of surviving. It is to be decided whether all HIV infected mothers

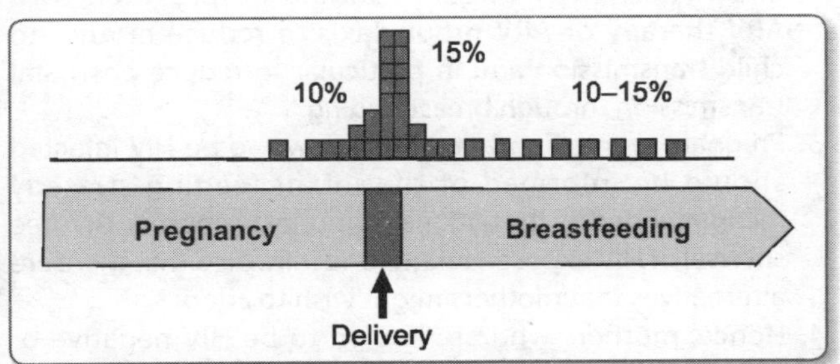

Fig. 17.1: HIV transmission risk before perinatal HIV prevention

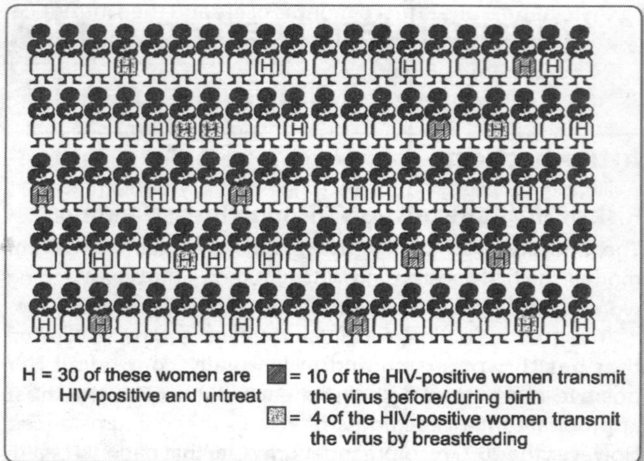

Fig. 17.2: Hundred women breastfeed where HIV is prevalent

will breastfeed and receive antiretroviral (ARV) injections or will avoid all breastfeeding.

1. Currently WHO is developing guidance to assist countries in this decision-making process and all steps to reach these standards of care. Whichever option is chosen, mothers should be helped and empowered to sustain that option.
2. Current WHO recommendations advocate that all mothers known to be HIV infected should be provided with ARV therapy or ARV prophylaxis to reduce mother to child transmission and in particular to reduce postnatal transmission through breastfeeding.
3. Pregnant women and mothers known to be HIV infected should be informed of the infant feeding strategy recommended by the national authority to improve HIV-free survival of HIV exposed infants and informed that there are alternatives that mothers might wish to adopt.
4. Hence, mothers who are known to be HIV negative or whose HIV status is known or infants of HIV positive mothers known to be HIV infected should exclusively breastfeed

their infants for the first 6 months of life and then introduce complementary foods, while continuing breastfeeding for 24 months or beyond.

5. HIV infected mothers on ARV therapy or prophylaxis (whose infants are HIV infected or known HIV status) should exclusively breastfeed those infants for the first 6 months of life, introducing appropriate complementary foods, thereafter, and continue breastfeeding for the first 12 months of life. Breastfeeding should then only stop once a nutritionally adequate and safe diet without breast milk can be provided. As per the new guidelines, baby should receive daily nevirapine from birth until 1 week after all exposure to breast milk has ended if the mother received only zidovudine prophylaxis and nevirapine from birth to 6 weeks if mother has received triple ARV prophylaxis.
6. The HIV positive mother not to breastfeed in spite of receiving ARV prophylaxis, zidovudine or nevirapine is indicated for 6 weeks for the baby from birth.
7. Whenever HIV infected mothers decide to stop breastfeeding, it should be done gradually within 1 month. Mothers or infants who have received ARV prophylaxis should continue for 1 week after breastfeeding is fully stopped.
8. Infants born to HIV infected women receiving antiretroviral therapy (ART) should receive daily nevirapine from birth till 6 weeks of age and for more being breastfed daily, zidovudine or nevirapine from birth until 6 weeks of age is recommended.

Alternatives of Breastfeeding

For Infants Less Than 6 Months of Age

- Expressed, heat-treated breast milk
- Unmodified animal milk
- Commercial infant formula milk.

The choice/selection shall be based on AFASS criteria.

For Children over 6 Months of Age

- All children can be given complementary foods from 6 months of age. Meals including, foods, combination of milk and other foods, should be provided.

Other Options for All Ages

- Breastfeeding by another woman who is HIV negative (wet-nursing)
- Human milk from breast milk banks.

Replacement Feeding

Replacement feeding (RF) is the process of feeding a child who is not receiving any breast milk, with a diet that provides all the nutrients until the child is fully fed on family food. The replacement feeding option should be selected, any if all of the acceptability, feasibility, affordability, safety and sustainability (AFASS) criteria are completely fulfilled. Cup feeding should be the method of choice if replacement feeding needs to be done and bottles should be totally avoided, if any of the AFASS criteria is not met, mother should practice exclusive breastfeeding till 6 months along with early treatment of breast and nipple problems of HIV positive mother.

Mothers known to be HIV infected may consider expressing and heat-treating breast milk as an interim feeding strategy in special circumstances such as:

- When the infant is born with LBW or is otherwise ill in the neonatal period and unable to breastfeed; or
- When the mother is unwell and temporarily unable to breastfeed or has a temporary breast health problem such as mastitis; or
- If ARV drugs are temporary not available.

chapter 18

Breastfeeding in Special Situations

Introduction

There are some breastfeeding challenges. These are special situations. They are not problems. Twins, cleft lip and palate, working mother, implants, pregnancy induced hypertension (PIH), adopting, mother sick, baby sick, yes you can do it. It may be a "challenge" but you can do it if (1) do not quit and (2) find a good support system.

Breastfed Twins

Best thing is to contact someone who has breastfed twins. Breastfeeding twins require more work, dedication, responsibility (Figs 18.1A and B). Mother may worry that she would not produce enough milk for two. Or she may be afraid that nursing twins will take too much time, common problems such as sore or cracked nipples, engorgement and low milk

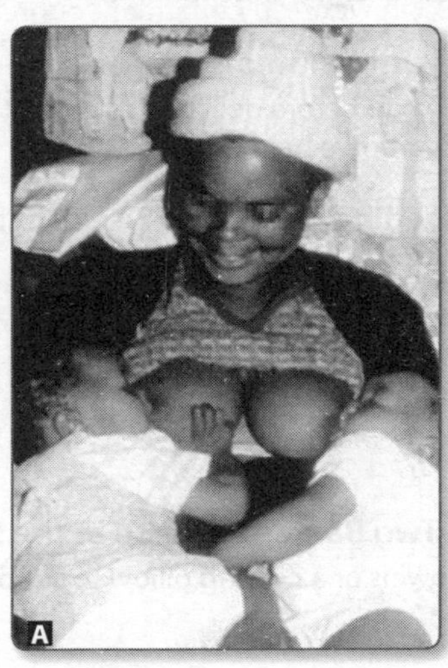
A

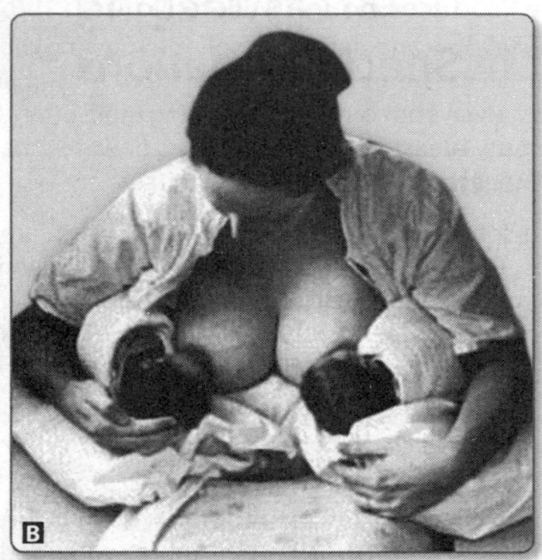

Figs 18.1A and B: (A and B) Breastfeeding twins

supply, and worry. Mother needs support from baby's doctor, lactation specialist, family and friend.

How to Deal with Common Challenges?

Knowing what to do before delivery is better. It will help ease her anxiety and prepare her for the job ahead.

Does Breastfeeding Take More Time Than Bottle Feeding?

No.

A Rigid Time Bound or Flexible Demand Feeding Schedule

Demand feeding.

How to Hold Two Babies to Nurse at the Same Time?

Use rolled up towels or a nursing pillow to support babies.

Can She Produce Enough Milk to Nourish Two?

The law of supply and demand applies to nursing mothers of twins. Trust in nature and confidence matters. A low milk supply can almost always be corrected by nursing more often. If babies do not empty breasts, express. Keep lots of water nearby. The oxytocin released can make her very thirsty.

How to Know If Babies Are Getting Enough Milk?

(1) Weight gain; (2) babies feeding at least 8 times a day; (3) at least three stools in a day; (3) they wet six or more diapers a day; (4) you can hear babies swallowing while nursing and (5) breasts feel softer after nursing.

The following drawings show various positioning ideas for twins (Figs 18.2A to F).

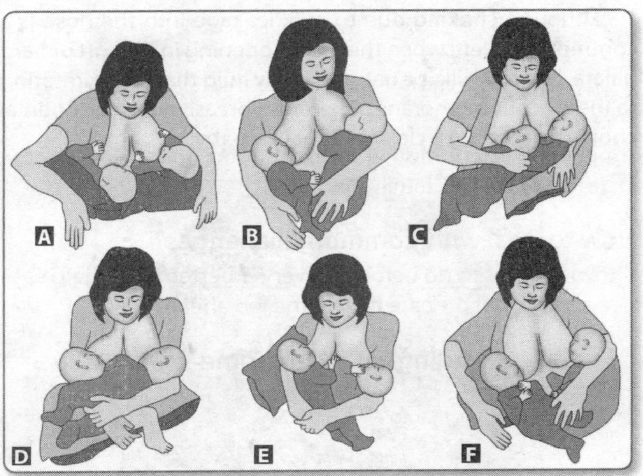

Figs 18.2A to F: (A to F) Various positions of ideas for twins

Breastfeeding A Cleft Lip/Palate Baby

Mother of a child with cleft lip/palate is shocked and worried (Fig. 18.3). She is not sure that she can manage such a child. These uncertainties can affect the early bonding phases of parenting.

Mother and baby should spend more time together. If breastfeeding is initiated right after birth, closeness between mother and baby will be enhanced. Mothers and babies find the skin to skin contact during breastfeeding calming and comforting.

The soft breast is ideal for the baby's mouth. The flexibility of the breast allows it to be moulded to compensate for abnormalities of the baby's lip or mouth. The baby has more control over the flow of milk and the position of the breast in his or her mouth. Early practice helps baby imprint on the breast.

Although choking due to milk leakage into the nose is a common problem when there is an opening in the soft or hard palate, human milk is a natural bodily fluid that is not irritating to the mucous membranes. Therefore, breast milk is the optimal choice for feeding a cleft lip or palate baby.

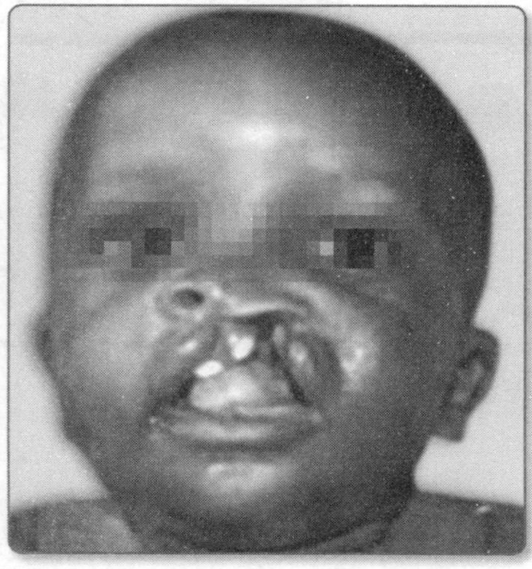

Fig. 18.3: A cleft lip/palate baby

A baby needs to suck for comfort as well as nourishment. Breastfeeding allows a baby to spend time at the breast sucking for comfort as well as for feeding.

Prior to the repair and possibly immediately after surgery, mother may find that they need to stimulate their milk supply by expressing it. Expressed milk can be fed to the baby by cup feeding. Lactation consultants (breastfeeding specialists) provide support and answer the questions. Breastfeeding early after surgical repair is encouraged. The goal is to make the surgical repair a positive experience by encouraging bonding, good nutrition and optimal growth for the child.

Breastfeeding and Working Mother

Work and breastfeeding can happen at the same time (Fig. 18.4). She can exclusively breastfeed her baby if she knows how to do it and she has a desire. A good start is important. Proper breastfeeding should be established in first 6 weeks. Success at expressing and storing is all that matters. She has to express and store every 2–3 hours, if she wants to exclusively (100%) breastfed. But no, if she is willing to supplement with some

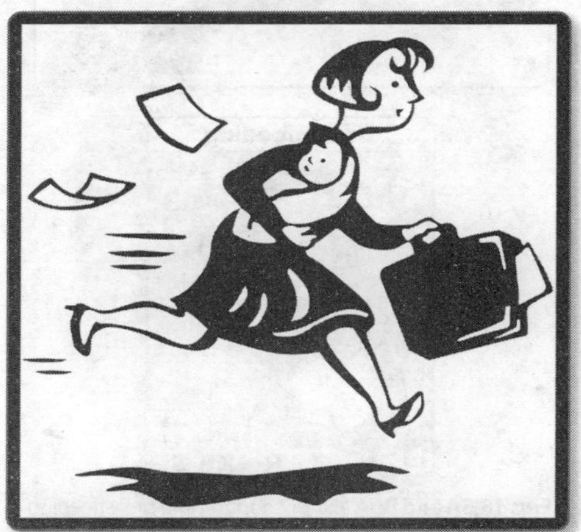

Fig. 18.4: Working mother

formula. It does not have to be all or nothing. Mother should ask for a 6-month breastfeeding leave, a place to express every 2–3 hours on job, a facility to store the expressed milk. Working and breastfeeding, it is worth it.

Adoption and Breastfeeding (Figs 18.5A and B)

A woman can produce breast milk without being pregnant. This is called as induced lactation. It is possible and has been successfully done by many women. Along with putting a baby to the breast. Birth control pills, domperidone, breast pump, diet and water are essential parts of relactation program. A strong desire is essential.

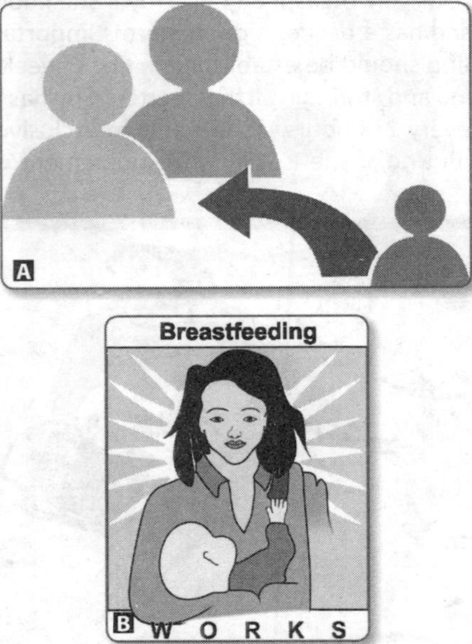

Figs 18.5A and B: (A and B) Adoption and breastfeeding

Tandem Nursing

Tandem nursing is the term used to describe breastfeeding an older child through pregnancy, then continuing to breastfeed both the older child and the newborn (Figs 18.6A and B). It is not necessary to wean off the older baby because mother has become pregnant again. Milk during pregnancy is not bad. If the mother takes adequate diet, she can breastfeed during pregnancy. She can breastfeed both babies, newborn and older.

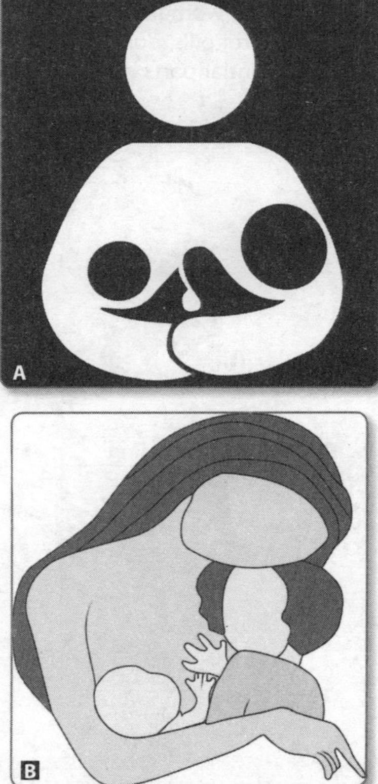

Figs 18.6A and B: (A and B) Tandem nursing

chapter 19

Infant Milk Substitutes Act

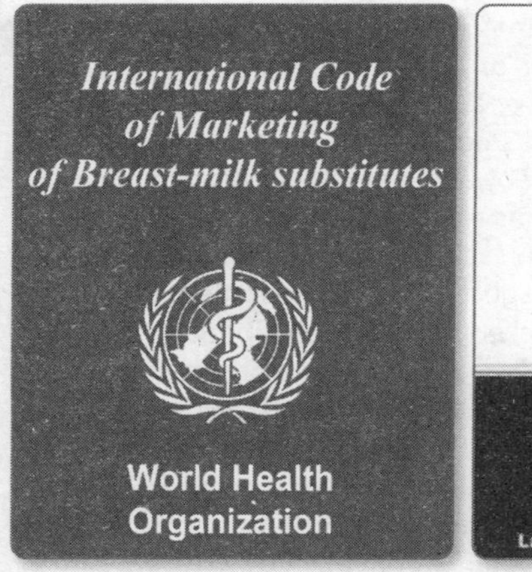

The Infant Milk Substitutes, Feeding Bottles and Infant Foods (Regulation of Production, Supply and Distribution) Act, 1992, as Amended in 2003 (IMS Act)

It provides for the regulation of production, supply and distribution of infant milk substitutes, feeding bottles and infant foods with a view to the protection and promotion of breastfeeding and ensuring the proper use of infant foods and for matters connected therewith or incidental thereto.

Be it enacted by Parliament in the 54th year of the Republic of India as follows:

1. (1) This act may be called the Infant Milk Substitutes, Feeding Bottles and Infant Foods (Regulation of Production, Supply and Distribution) Act, 1992, as amended in 2003 (IMS Act).

(2) It extends to the whole of India.

(3) It shall come into force on such date as Central Government may, by notification in the Official Gazette, appoint.

2. (1) In this Act, unless the context otherwise requires,

(a) "advertisement" includes any notice, circular, label, wrapper or any other document or visible representation or announcement made by means of any light, sound, smoke or gas or by means of electronic transmission or by audio or visual transmission;

(b) "container" means a box, bottle, casket, tin, can, barrel, case, receptacle, sack, wrapper or other thing in which any infant milk substitute, feeding bottle or infant food is placed or packed for sale or distribution;

(c) "feeding bottle" means ant bottle or receptacle used for purpose of feeding infant milk substitutes, and includes a teat and a valve attached are capable of being attached to such bottle or receptacle;

(d) "health care system" means an institution or organization engaged, either directly or indirectly, in health care for mothers, infants or pregnant women, and includes a health workers in private practice, a pharmacy, drug store and any association of health workers;

(e) "health worker" means a person engaged in health care for mothers, infants or pregnant women;

(f) "infant food" means any food (by whatever name called) being marketed or otherwise represented as a complement to mother's milk to meet the growing nutritional needs of the infant after the age of 6 months and up to the age of 2 years;

(g) "infant milk substitute" means any food being marketed or otherwise represented as a partial or total replacement for mother's milk, for infant up to the age of 2 years;

(h) "label" means a display of written, marked, stamped, printed or graphed matter affixed to, or appearing upon, any container;

(i) "prescribed" means prescribed by rules made under this Act;

(j) "promotion" means to employ directly or indirectly any method of encouraging any person to purchase or use infant milk substitute, feeding bottle or infant food.

(2) Any reference in this Act to any other enactment or any provision thereof, shall, in relation to an area in which such enactment or such provision is not in force, be constructed as a reference to the corresponding law or the relevant provision of the corresponding law, if any, in force in that area.

3. No person shall

(a) advertise, or take part in the publication of any advertisement, for the distribution, sale or supply of infant milk substitutes, feeding bottles or infant foods; or

(b) give an impression or create a belief in any manner that feeding of infant milk substitutes and infant foods are equivalent to, or better than, mother's milk; or

(c) take part in the promotion of infant milk substitutes, feeding bottles or infant foods.

4. No person shall

(a) supply or distribute samples of infant milk substitutes or feeding bottles or infant foods or gifts of utensils or other articles; or

(b) contact any pregnant women or the mother of an infant; or

(c) offer inducement of any other kind.

For the purpose of promoting the use or sale of infant milk substitutes or feeding bottles or infant foods.

5. Subject to the provisions of subsection (4) of section 8, no person shall donate or distribute

(a) infant milk substitutes or feeding bottles or infant foods to any other person except to an orphanage;

(b) any informational or educational equipment or material relating to infant milk substitutes or feeding bottles or infant foods:

Provided that nothing in this clause shall apply to the donation or distribution, subject to such conditions and restrictions as may be prescribed, of such equipment or material through the health care system.

6. (1) Without prejudice to the provisions of the Prevention of Food Adulteration Act, 1954 and the rules made thereunder, no person shall produce, supply or distribute any infant milk substitute or infant food unless every container thereof or any label affixed thereto indicates in a clear, conspicuous and in an easily readable and understandable manner, the words "important notice" in capital letters in such language as may be prescribed and indicating thereunder the following particulars in the same language, namely:

(a) a statement "mother's milk is best for your baby" in capital letters;
(b) a statement that infant milk substitute or infant food should be used only on the advice of a health worker as to the need for its use and the proper method of its use;
(c) a warning that infant milk substitute or infant food is not the sole source of nourishment of an infant;
(d) the instructions for its appropriate preparation and a warning against the health hazards of its inappropriate preparation;
(e) the ingredients used ;
(f) the composition or analysis;
(g) the storage conditions required;
(h) the batch number, date of its manufacture and the date before which it is to be consumed, taking into account the climatic and storage conditions of the country;
(i) such other particulars as may be prescribed.

(2) No container or label referred to in subsection (1) relating to infant milk substitute or infant food shall

(a) have pictures of an infant or a women or both; or
(b) have pictures or other graphic material or phrases designed to increase the salability of infant milk substitutes or infant food; or

(c) use on it the word "humanized" or "maternalized" or any other similar word ; or

(d) bear on it such other particulars as may be prescribed.

7. (1) Every educational or other material including advertisements or material relating to promotion of infant milk substitutes, feeding bottles and infant foods whether audio or visual, dealing with prenatal or postnatal care or with the feeding of an infant and intended to reach pregnant women or mothers of infants shall include clear information relating to

(a) the benefits and superiority of breastfeeding;

(b) the preparation for, and the continuance of, breastfeeding;

(c) the harmful effects on breastfeeding due to the partial adoption of bottle feeding;

(d) the difficulties in reverting to breastfeeding of infants after a period of feeding by infant milk substitute;

(e) the financial and social implications in making use of infant milk substitutes and feeding bottles;

(f) the health hazards of improper use of infant milk substitutes and feeding bottles;

(g) the date of printing and publication of such material and the name of the printer and publisher;

(h) such other matters as may be prescribed.

8. (1) No person shall use any health care system for the display of placards or posters relating to, or for the distribution of, materials for the purpose of promoting the use or sale of infant milk substitutes or feeding bottles or infant foods:

Provided that the provisions of this subsection shall not apply to

(a) the donation or distribution of informational or educational equipment or material made in accordance with the proviso to clause (b) of section 5; and

(b) the dissemination of information to a health worker about the scientific and factual matters relating to the use of infant milk substitutes or feeding bottles or infant foods along with the information specified in subsection (1) of section 7.

(2) No person who produces, supplies, distributes or sells infant milk substitutes or feeding bottles or infant foods shall make any payment to any person who works in the health care system for the purpose of promoting the use or sale of such substitutes or bottles or foods.

(3) No person, other than a health worker, shall demonstrate feeding with infant milk substitutes or infant foods to a mother of an infant or to any member of her family and such health worker shall also clearly explain to such mother or such other member the hazards of improper use of infant milk substitutes or feeding bottles or infant foods.

(4) No person, other than an institution or organization, engaged in health care for mothers, infants or pregnant women, shall distribute infant milk substitutes or feeding bottles to a mother who cannot resort to breastfeeding and who cannot afford to purchase infant milk substitutes or feeding bottles.

(5) An orphanage may purchase infant milk substitutes or feeding bottles at a price lower than their sale price for the purpose of utilizing them in the said orphanage.

Explanation: For the purposes of this subsection, such purchases shall not amount to an inducement for promoting the use or sale of infant milk substitutes or feeding bottles.

9. (1) No person who produces, distributes or sells infant milk substitutes or feeding bottles or infant foods shall offer or give, directly or indirectly, any financial inducements or gifts to a health worker or to any member of his family for the purpose of promoting the use of such substitutes or bottles or foods.

(2) No producer, supplier or distributor referred to in subsection (1), shall offer or give any contribution or pecuniary benefit to a health worker or any association of health workers, including funding of seminar, meeting, conferences, educational course, contest, fellowship, research work of sponsorship.

10. (1) No person who produces, supplies, distributes or sells infant milk substitutes or feeding bottles or infant foods shall fix the remuneration of any of his employees or give any commission to such employees on the basis of the volume of sale of such substitutes or bottles or foods made by such employees.

(2) The employees of such person shall not perform any function which relates to educating a pregnant woman or mother of an infant on prenatal or postnatal care of the infant.

11. (1) No person shall sell or otherwise distribute any infant milk substitute or infant food unless it conforms to the standards, specified for such substitute or food under the Prevention of Food Adulteration Act, 1954, and the rules made thereunder and the container thereof has the relevant Standard Mark specified by the Bureau of India Standards established under section 3 of the Bureau of Indian Standards Act, 1986 to indicate that the infant milk substitutes or infant food conforms to such standards:

Provided that where no standards have been specified for any infant milk substitute or infant food under the Prevention of food Adulteration Act, 1954, no person shall sell or otherwise distribute such substitute food unless he has obtained the approval of the Central Government in relation to such substitute or food and the label affixed to the container thereof under the rules made under that Act.

(2) No person shall sell or otherwise distribute any feeding bottle unless it conforms to the Standard Mark specified by the Bureau of Indian Standards referred to in subsection (1) for feeding bottles and such mark is affixed on its container.

12. (1) Any food inspector appointed under section 9 of the Prevention of Food Adulteration Act, 1954 (hereinafter referred to as the food inspector) or any officer not below the rank of a Class 1 officer authorized in this behalf by the State Government (hereinafter referred to as the authorized officer) may, if he has any reason to believe that any provision of section 6 or section 11 has been or is being

contravened. Enter and search, at any reasonable time, any factory, building, business premises or any other place where any trade or commerce in infant milk substitutes or feeding bottles or infant foods is carried on or such substitutes or bottles or foods are produced, supplied or distributed.

(2) The Provisions of the Code of Criminal Procedure, 1973, relating to searches and seizures shall, so far as may be, apply to every search or seizure made under this Act.

13. (1) If any food inspector or authorized officer has reason to believe that in respect of any infant milk substitute or feeding bottle or infant food or container thereof, the provisions of this Act have been or are being contravened, he may seize such substitute or bottle or food or container.

(2) No such substitute or food or bottle or container shall be retained by any food inspector or authorized officer for a period exceeding 90 days from the date of its seizure unless the approval of the District Judge, within the local limits of whose jurisdiction such seizure has been made, has been obtained for such retention.

14. Any infant milk substitute or feeding bottle or infant food or container thereof, in respect of which any provision of this Act has been or is being contravened, shall be liable to confiscation:

Provided that where it is established to the satisfaction of the court adjudging the confiscation that the person in whose possession, power or control any such substitute or bottle or food or container is found is not responsible for the contravention of the provisions of this Act, the court may, instead of making an order for the confiscation of such substitute or bottle or food or container, make such other order authorized by this Act against the person guilty of the breach of the provisions of this Act as it may think fit.

15. (1) Whenever any confiscation is authorized by this Act the court adjudging it may, subject to such conditions as may be specified in the order adjudging the confiscation, give to the owner thereof an option to pay in lieu of

confiscation such cost not exceeding the value of the infant milk substitute or feeding bottle or infant food or container thereof in respect of which the confiscation is authorized as the court thinks fit.

(2) On payment of the cost ordered by the court the seized infant milk substitute or feeding bottle or container shall be returned to the person from whom it was seized on the condition that such person shall, before making any distribution, sale or supply of such substitute or bottle or food or container, give effect to the provisions of this Act.

16. No confiscation made or cost ordered to be paid under this Act shall prevent the infliction of any punishment to which the person affected thereby is liable under the provisions of this Act or under any other law.

17. Any confiscation may be adjudged or costs may be ordered to be paid:

(a) without any limit, by the principal civil court of original jurisdiction within the local limits of whose jurisdiction such confiscation has been made or costs have been ordered to be paid, as the case may be;

(b) subject to such limits as may be specified by the Central Government in this behalf, by such other court, not below a civil court having pecuniary jurisdiction exceeding 5,000 rupees, as the Central Government may, by notification in the Official Gazette, authorize in this behalf.

18. (1) No order adjudicating confiscation or directing payment of costs shall be made unless the owner of the infant milk substitute or feeding bottle or infant food or container thereof has been given a notice in writing informing him of the grounds on which it is proposed to confiscate such substitute or bottle or container and giving him a reasonable opportunity of making a representation in writing, within such reasonable time as may be specified in the notice, against the confiscation and if he so desires, of being heard in the matter:

Provided that where no such notice is given within a period of 90 days from the date of the seizure of the infant milk substitute or feeding bottle or infant food or container thereof, such substitute or bottle or food or container shall be returned after the expiry of that period to the person from whose possession it was seized.

(2) Save as otherwise provided in subsection (1), the provisions of the Code of Civil Procedure, 1908, shall, so far as may be, apply to every proceeding referred to in subsection (1).

19. (1) Any person aggrieved by any decision of the court adjudication a confiscation or ordering the payment of costs may prefer an appeal to the court to which an appeal lies from the decision of such court.

(2) The appellate court may, after giving the appellant an opportunity of being heard, pass such order as it thinks fit confirming, modifying or revising the decision or order appealed against or may send back the case with such directions as it may think fit for a fresh decision or adjudication, as the case may be, after taking additional evidence if necessary:

Provided that an order enhancing any fine in lieu of confiscation or for confiscating goods of greater value shall not be made under this section unless the appellant has had an opportunity of making a representation and if he so desires of being heard in his defense.

(3) No further appeal shall lie against the order of the court made under subsection (2).

20. (1) Any person who contravenes the provisions of section 3, 4, 5, 7, 8, 9, 10 or subsection (2) of section 11 and the rules made under section 26 of the Act shall be punishable with imprisonment for a term which may extend to 3 years, or with fine which may extend to 5,000 rupees, or with both.

(2) Any person who contravenes the provisions of section 6 or subsection (1) of section 11 and the rules made under section 26 of the Act shall be punishable with imprisonment for a term which shall not be less than 6 months but which may extend to 3 years and with fine which shall not be less than 2,000 rupees.

Provided that the court may, for any adequate and special reasons to be mentioned in the judgment, impose a sentence of imprisonment for 44 Law 2, a term which shall not be less than 3 months but which may extend to 2 years and with fine which shall not be less than 1,000 rupees.

21. (1) Save as otherwise provided in section 173 of the Code of Criminal Procedure, 1973, no court shall take cognizance of any offence punishable under this Act except upon a complaint in writing made by

(a) a person authorized in this behalf under subsection (1) of section 20 of the Prevention of Food Adulteration Act, 1954; or

(b) an officer not below the rank of a Class 1 officer authorized in this behalf, by general or special order, by the Government; or

(c) a representative of such voluntary organization engaged in the field of child welfare and development and child nutrition as the Government may, by notification in the Official Gazette, authorize in this behalf.

(2) Where a complaint has been made by a representative of the voluntary organization authorized under clause (c) of subsection (1) and the court has issued a summons or, as the case may be, a warrant under subsection (1) of section 204 of the Code of Criminal Procedure, 1973, the Assistant Public Prosecutor for that court shall take charge of the case and conduct the prosecution.

22. (1) Where an offence under this Act has been committed by a company, every person who, at the time the offence was committed, was in charge of, and was responsible to, the company for the conduct of the business of the company, as well as the company, shall be deemed to be guilty of the offence and shall be liable to be proceeded against and punished accordingly:

Provided that nothing contained in this subsection shall render any such person liable to any punishment, if the proves that the offence was committed without his knowledge or that he had exercised all due diligence to prevent the commission of such offence.

(2) Notwithstanding anything contained in subsection (1), where any offence under this Act has been committed by a company and it is proved that the offence has been committed with the consent or connivance of, or it attributable to any neglect on the part of, any director, manager, secretary or other officer of the company, such director, manager, secretary or other officer shall also be deemed to be guilty of that offence and shall be liable to be proceeded against and punished accordingly.

Explanation: For the purposes of this section,

(a) "company" means any body corporate and includes a firm or other association of individuals; and

(b) "director", in relation to a firm, means a partner in the firm.

23. Notwithstanding anything contained in the Code of Criminal Procedure, 1973, an offence punishable under this Act shall be

(a) bailable;

(b) cognizable.

24. No suit, prosecution or other legal proceeding shall lie against the Central Government or any State Government or any officer of the Central Government or a representative of such voluntary organization which is notified under clause (c) of subsection (1) of section 21 for anything which is in good faith done or intended to be done under this Act.

25. The provisions of this Act, or the rules made thereunder shall be in addition to, and not in derogation of, the Prevention of Food Adulteration Act, 1954, or the rules made thereunder.

26. (1) The Central Government may, by notification in the Official Gazette, make rules to carryout the provisions of this Act.

(2) In particular, and without prejudice to the generality of the foregoing power, such rules may provide for all or any of the following matters, namely:

(a) the conditions and restrictions subject to which educational equipment and other material may be donated or distributed under the provision to clause (b) of section 5;

(b) the language in which the notice and other particulars shall be indicated under subsection (1) of section 6;

(c) the particulars which are to be indicated under clause (i) of subsection (1) of section 6;

(d) the particulars which a container or label shall not bear under clause (d) of subsection (2) of section 6;

(e) the matters to be included in the information which reaches pregnant women or mothers of infants under clause (g) of subsection (1) of section 7;

(f) any other matter which is required to be, or may be, prescribed.

(3) Every rule made under this Act shall be laid, as soon as may be after it is made, before each House of Parliament, while it is in section, for a total period of 30 days which may be comprised in one session or in two or more successive sessions, and if, before the expiry of the session immediately following the session or the successive sessions aforesaid, both Houses agree in making any modification in the rule or both Houses agree that the rule should not be made, the rule shall thereafter have effect only in such modified form or be of no effect, as the case may be; so, however, that any such modification or annulment shall be without prejudice to the validity of anything previously done under that rule.

Bibliography

1. Baby Breastfeeding within Minutes after Birth
   http://www.youtube.com/watch?v=dLboKrCeVOA&feature=related
2. Breastfeeding a Cleft Child
   http://www.youtube.com/watch?v=404ciRmmZas&feature=related
3. Breastfeeding
   http://www.youtube.com/watch?v=TxbvJ9eu21A&feature=related
4. Breastfeeding in Public (Australian Breastfeeding Association Advert)
   http://www.youtube.com/watch?v=VnReJeQrK0k&feature=player_embedded#t=29s
5. Breastfeeding in Public
   http://www.youtube.com/watch?v=rrnxtiYmXig&NR=1
6. Breastfeeding—Baby Led Mother Guided Started Upright Left Breast, Latches
   http://www.youtube.com/watch?v=UYcpkYrOPBE&feature=related
7. Breastfeeding—Cradle Hold
   http://www.youtube.com/watch?v=mbkw9Yrqa3g&feature=related
8. Breasts Are the BEST!
   http://www.youtube.com/watch?v=zXOVO4rc7mo&NR=1&feature=fvwp
9. English—Initiation of Breastfeeding by Breast Crawl
   http://www.youtube.com/watch?v=b3oPb4WdycE&feature=related
10. How to Breastfeed: How to Breastfeed in Public
    http://www.youtube.com/watch?v=iUG5cW6rzas&feature=related
11. How to Breastfeed: How to Breastfeed in the Car
    http://www.youtube.com/watch?v=6YjMC1w2bJA&feature=related

12. How to Breastfeed Your Baby Safely! Free Breastfeeding Advice Breastfeeding Education
http://www.youtube.com/watch?v=UVXx3128xsU&NR=1
13. Infant Nutritional Care: How to Breastfeed Twins
http://www.youtube.com/watch?v=U8kj8L-A_QQ

Index

Page numbers followed by *f* refer to figure